THE SOUTH BEACH DIET DINING GUIDE

Arthur Agatston, MD

Author of the *New York Times* Bestseller *The South Beach Diet*

RODALE

© 2005 by Arthur Agatston, MD

Book design by Carol Angstadt

ISBN-13 978-1-59486-360-8 paperback

ISBN-10 1-59486-360-1 paperback

Distributed to the trade by Holtzbrinck Publishers

2 4 6 8 10 9 7 5 3 1 paperback

CONTENTS

FOREWORD

Americans spend $440 billion eating out at restaurants each year. And every day, one in four Americans eats fast food. These statistics are hardly surprising. We work hard. We're constantly on the go, whether it's carpooling our kids from school to a sports match or traveling for business. But while dining out may provide a convenient, time-saving solution to a hectic lifestyle, it also presents a troubling scenario.

Today, according to the most recent statistics from the Centers for Disease Control, an estimated 64 percent of American adults age 20 years or older are considered overweight or obese. The cause of this epidemic is too much processed, nutrient- and fiber-poor food. The fact is, while Americans are overfed, we are actually undernourished. This is true of American adults and especially true of our children. We are undernourished because we are not getting the vast array of nutrients found in the good carbs and the good fats that are essential for prevention of heart disease, cancer, and other diseases of Western society. We also need these nutrients for our optimal day-to-day functioning because we all feel better when we eat better.

The good news is that an increasing number of busy Americans do want to incorporate better nutrition into their everyday lives. Because educated consumers have been effectively expressing their desire for healthier foods, there is already a clear movement in the restaurant industry to accommodate healthy eaters. Recently McDonald's announced that it will print dietary information, including calories, fat, protein, carbohydrates, and sodium, on its food wrappers. Other chains are sure to follow. In addition, many fast-casual restaurants are now striving to provide healthier food choices, from grilled chicken and fresh steamed vegetables to whole-grain breads for take-out sandwiches. These are wonderful trends that I believe will continue as Americans become more aware of the principles of a healthy diet.

It's because eating out is such an integral part of American life that we decided to create *The South Beach Diet Dining Guide*. We wanted to make it easy for you as an individual or as a family to navigate this often complicated and challenging world, whether you're eating fast food or fancy food, whether you're waiting at the airport, enjoying a ballgame, or dining out for business. The truth is, there are almost always healthy choices to be made wherever you dine—and certainly some pitfalls to be avoided. This book will teach you what they are so that you can maintain your South Beach Diet lifestyle and never feel deprived.

In this handy, pocket-size guide, we've included more than 75 chain and family restaurants, from Applebee's to Whataburger, as well as 75 business-class restaurants in 15 of the most traveled cities from coast to coast. Our goal is to provide you with the information you'll need to make the best possible choice of restaurant—and then to make the best possible food choices at that restaurant. While we certainly don't recommend tacos, pizza, or hamburgers as South Beach Diet fare, we know that there will be times when eating this type of fast food is unavoidable. Therefore, we've given you what we think are the best choices in such chains. We've also made an effort to list only those dishes that a South Beach dieter can eat along with the appropriate phase. If you don't see one of your favorite (seemingly healthy) menu items listed for a popular restaurant, it's probably because we were surprised to discover that it contained hidden sugar, fat, or starch, and we decided not to include it in this book.

No matter where you're dining, I urge you to discuss the food preparation with your server. You may be able to have a particular menu item prepared without high-fat sauces, croutons, or dressings. In fact, while researching this book, we learned that P.F. Chang's China Bistro will gladly stir-fry a dish in broth—if you ask. And Burger King will serve a burger bunless—if you ask. Even in fancy restaurants, like those included in our Business Dining section, you shouldn't feel shy about making your South Beach Diet preferences known. We know from talking to these restaurants that they will be more than happy to accommodate you.

Clearly, consumer awareness about healthy eating has encouraged change in the restaurant industry. After years of confusion experienced not just by the public but also by health-care professionals, there is finally a consensus on the principles of healthy eating. We have moved beyond the low fat versus low carb debates and have come to agree that our focus should be on nutrient-dense, fiber-rich foods, healthy sources of unsaturated fats, and lean sources of protein. We have also learned a great deal more about how important these guidelines are to our general health, not just to our waistlines. In fact, even if you have no weight to lose, you should still be following these recommendations.

As I've said before, the challenge is in incorporating this knowledge into everyday life. The bottom line is that if we do not make better food choices, then our obesity rate will continue to increase as our health deteriorates and our medical-care costs skyrocket. With *The South Beach Diet Dining Guide,* we hope to advance our goal of changing the way America eats.

Arthur Agatston, MD

DINING OUT
ON THE SOUTH BEACH DIET

You have a busy life. Chances are that work and family keep you on the go, and preparing home-cooked meals may be difficult because of time constraints. Finding a healthy lunch in the middle of a hectic day is often just as hard, and eating a good breakfast at home may be a rare event. In fact, if you're like most Americans, you purchase at least one meal a day at some sort of restaurant.

And that's just on an ordinary day. What about weekends, holidays, special occasions, travel days, business dinners, and all the other times you're away from your own kitchen? Does this mean putting your South Beach Diet on hold?

Not at all.

One of the best things about the South Beach Diet is that it's easy to dine out—and still eat well—while following the principles of the program. No matter what phase you're on, you can continue to lose weight and improve your health, whether you're grabbing a take-out order or enjoying dinner with family, friends, or business associates at a fine restaurant.

The first, and most important, step in sticking to the South Beach Diet when eating out is to keep the following ground rules in mind:

- Choose unprocessed, unrefined carbohydrates, such as whole grains, whole fruits, and fresh vegetables.
- Enjoy plenty of lean protein, such as chicken, fish, certain cuts of meat, low-fat dairy, and reduced-fat cheese.
- Choose foods that are high in good fats, such as fish, avocados, and nuts, and make sure your foods are prepared with healthy oils such as olive oil or canola.

- Avoid foods that are high in saturated fat, such as fatty cuts of beef, bacon, processed meats such as salami, and full-fat cheese.
- Eat plenty of fiber—it's found in fruits, vegetables, nuts, beans, seeds, and whole grains.
- Avoid refined carbohydrates such as white bread, cake, candy, white rice, and other processed foods that are high in sugar and often high in fat as well.
- Avoid added sugar. Choose diet soft drinks, for instance, and watch out for hidden sugars in salad dressings and sauces.

Once you have the ground rules down, you'll also need to master some proven strategies that will help you enjoy your restaurant meals even more.

Key Strategies for Restaurant Dining

Dining out is one of life's pleasures, but it's also a challenge when you're trying to maintain a healthy diet. At home you can control what you put on your plate, but when you eat out, you're bound to come up against some common pitfalls: oversized portions, tempting refined carbs, extra ingredients that add bad fat and bad carbs, and of course menus that don't offer many South Beach Diet–friendly options. The following tips will help you stick to your healthy eating plan.

• **Have a protein snack before you leave the house.** By eating something with protein—a hard-boiled egg or a piece of reduced-fat cheese, for example—about 15 minutes before you arrive at the restaurant, you'll take the edge off your appetite. If you're not ravenous while you're reading the menu, you'll be able to make better food choices.

• **Banish the bread basket.** And the tortilla chips basket. And the crispy noodle basket. They're all filled with bad (refined) carbs, such as rolls made from white flour or deep-fried tortilla chips. Eating these carbs will give you a glucose jolt that could raise your blood sugar, and you might end up feeling hungrier. If it's okay with your fellow diners, ask your server to remove the basket before you even have a chance to nibble. If not, wait until everyone has taken some and then ask the server to remove the basket. (If that's not appropriate for the group you're with, at least position the basket as far from yourself as possible.) Once you're on Phase 2 or 3, you can indulge in a slice from the bread basket—as long as it is made from whole grains. To prevent a rapid rise in blood sugar, dip the bread into olive oil or even spread a little butter on it. The added calories are offset by the feeling of fullness that the fat adds.

• **Order soup.** If possible, order a cup of soup—the dieter's friend—as soon as you're seated. Look for soups that are rich in vegetables and that aren't cream-based, or order clear broth or consommé. The beauty of soup is that it fills you up, so you're not so hungry when it comes time to order from the rest of the menu. It also sends a message to your brain that you're eating and will be full soon. Since it takes about 20 minutes for that message to travel from your stomach to your brain, by the time your main course arrives, you'll already be on the way to feeling satiated.

• **Ask for extra veggies instead of starches.** Main courses usually come with starchy side dishes, such as white rice or mashed potatoes, which are undesirable foods for South Beach dieters on Phase 1 and 2. Ask instead for extra green vegetables, such as broccoli or string beans, or for a small green salad. Today, this is a routine request in many restaurants—and your server should be happy to help.

• **Pick healthy cooking methods.** Stay away from anything on the menu that appears to be coated or battered and fried. If the dish comes with a rich butter or cheese sauce, ask for it on the side. Stick to cooking methods—such as roasting, broiling, baking, grilling, steaming, and even sautéing—that don't add bad fats.

• **Have a (nonalcoholic) drink or two.** When your server asks if you want something from the bar, order a glass of water or diet soda. Sip it instead of a mixed drink or beer, and order another to go with your meal. Beyond Phase 1, have a glass of red or white wine along with your food—this is a form of alcohol that's not only acceptable but good for you.

• **Enjoy dessert—within reason.** The South Beach Diet is a lifestyle, and life without dessert would be no fun at all! But you have to make the right choices. Skip high-fat, high-sugar desserts. After Phase 1, if the menu offers fresh fruit, like berries or melon, that's your best choice. If you decide to indulge in something more decadent, use common sense. Ask the server to bring extra forks, limit yourself to three bites, and then share the rest with your fellow diners. After you've been on the South Beach Diet for a while, you may well find that your sweet tooth is more than satisfied with a small portion.

Casual Dining

The average American eats in a chain restaurant specializing in fast food at least once a week. What's wrong with the food at these casual quick-serve restaurants? A lot. Let's start with the fact that the emphasis at most chains is on big, sweet, fat, and

Estimating Portion Size

Portions in restaurants have ballooned over the past couple of decades. Though on the South Beach Diet you should eat until you feel satiated, eating two or three times a normal serving of food means you could be getting a lot more calories, fat, and carbohydrates from your restaurant meal than you realize—and you may keep eating even after you're full simply because it's there. Use these simple tricks to eyeball your portions and get an idea of how oversized they really are:

• 3½ ounces of meat, fish, or poultry is about the size of a deck of cards or a computer mouse.

• 8 ounces of meat, fish, or poultry is roughly the size of a thin paperback book.

• 1 cup of brown rice or whole-wheat pasta is about the size of a tennis ball.

• A small roll is about the size of a small pack of tissues.

• 2 tablespoons of salad dressing is 1 ounce, or ⅛ of a cup—enough to fill one compartment in an ice-cube tray.

fast. There's no denying that most fast food is typically high in calories, saturated fats (from the meats and cooking oil), trans fats, and refined carbohydrates (from all those buns, pizza crusts, and french fries) and low in fiber (think pickle slice). That means you're getting a faster rise in blood sugar from the bad carbs— one that's not offset by any fiber. The overall effect of this can leave you feeling unsatisfied by your meal. So, while you're still in the restaurant, you end up ordering more food—usually a dessert high in refined carbs and fat—just to feel full. And even if you do feel full, the sensation probably won't last, and you'll be on the lookout for a snack just an hour or two later.

As a South Beach dieter, you obviously know that it's best to avoid quick-serve restaurants whenever possible. We do live in a fast-food world, however, and realistically speaking, you're going to end up in one of these places now and then. Luckily, there are South Beach Diet solutions that will still let you make good choices among the menu options at most chain and family restaurants, whether it's a hamburger, chicken, or pizza restaurant, a cafeteria, or a Mexican eatery.

Hamburger Restaurants

There are more than 12,000 McDonald's restaurants in the United States, over 8,000 Burger Kings, and over 6,000 Wendy's, to say nothing of all the other burger chains. They're everywhere—and that makes them hard to avoid, especially when you're in a hurry. The good news is that today just about all hamburger restaurants have made an effort to accommodate people who are trying to follow a healthy eating plan. Instead of a cheeseburger on a bun with special sauce, you can now easily ask for a bunless burger on a plate, without the sauce and the ketchup. You can even get a side salad instead of those tempting high-fat fries.

What's in Your Fast Food?

Almost all fast-food chain restaurants now provide detailed nutritional information about their food on their Web sites, including calorie counts, amounts of fat and saturated fat, carbohydrates, and fiber; some chains will soon be providing the nutritionals on the packaging. You can usually find out exactly what's in the standard menu items, although "limited-time" and "seasonal" offerings aren't always there. In addition, many of the chain Web sites now offer nutrition calculators that let you put together an imaginary meal and see precisely what it comes out to in terms of nutrients. The next time you get a hankering for a late-night fast-food meal, try using the nutritional calculator first. It will help you make the wisest decision about what to eat when you arrive at the restaurant.

But keep in mind that even a bunless burger is still potentially high in saturated fat and should be avoided if there are better choices available. Fortunately, many burger restaurants now offer meal–size salads topped with grilled chicken or shrimp. If you order one of these, be sure to skip the croutons or Parmesan toasts, and take care with the salad dressings—many are loaded with added sugar. As far as drinks go, avoid the supersized shakes and sugary sodas; choose diet soda, coffee, or water instead.

Chicken Chains

At most quick-serve chicken restaurants, fried chicken is the main attraction. Watch out for all the ways this type of restaurant can try to sell you fried chicken by calling it something else, like crispy, crunchy, coated, nugget, or popcorn. And that's not all that's fried: The chicken is generally accompanied by your choice of french fries, fried onion rings, fried zucchini sticks, or fried mozzarella sticks.

Luckily, at just about all the chicken chains, grilled chicken breasts are now on the menu in one way or another. And some places, like Boston Market, are adding rotisserie chicken to their offerings. You can usually get a grilled chicken Caesar salad or ask for a green salad to go under or with your grilled or rotisserie chicken. At some franchises you can even get a green vegetable such as string beans to round out your meal.

There may be times, however, when you're just stuck with the fried chicken. In that case, simply pull off and discard as much of the coating as you can.

Pizza Places

According to pizza industry sources, the average American eats 46 slices of pizza a year. As a South Beach dieter, you're not in this camp, but you can still occasionally enjoy your pizza if you're on Phase 2 or 3. Just do it the healthier way. Almost all chain pizza restaurants now offer a thin-crust option, which cuts back on the amount of refined carbs you get from a slice. Most also make a veggie pizza, which means you get good vegetables like green peppers and mushrooms while avoiding the saturated fats from pepperoni, sausage, and other full-fat meat toppings (although you could add some grilled chicken if the chain offers it). Keep in mind that even thin-crust pizza has its drawbacks: the high fat content of the mozzarella cheese (you can ask for less cheese on your order) and the sugar that's sometimes added to the tomato sauce. Some more upscale pizza chains like Uno Chicago Grill now offer sirloin steak and steamed or roasted veggies as menu options.

So order a slice of thin-crust veggie pizza and ask for a side salad—most pizza chains offer them now. But stay away from all the other side offerings, such as chicken wings, breadsticks, cheese sticks, cinnamon sticks, and anything that comes with a dipping sauce.

Mexican Fast Food

Mexican food is perhaps the fastest growing area of fast-food chains. While Mexican dishes do offer a change from hamburgers, when they're prepared American style (which means an abundance of bad fats), they can still be a challenge to South Beach dieters.

A lot of the newer quick-serve Mexican chains are sit-down, and you'll have to immediately pass up the deep-fried tortilla chips that arrive at your table even before you order. At these places and at others like Taco Bell and Del Taco that offer drive-thru, you'll have to resist ordering the tacos, burritos, quesadillas, and chimichangas (deep-fried flour tortillas filled with meat and cheese). That's unless you can get them "bare" or "naked," which means ordering the filling without the flour or corn tortilla. (If you're on Phase 2, a whole-wheat tortilla is allowed.) Best to stick to the grilled items, such as chicken, shrimp, or steak. You can also enjoy the pinto beans and black beans, but skip the fat-laden refried beans and the rice.

The good news is that fresh salsa is a highly acceptable SBD condiment, and guacamole is a great source of good fat from the avocados. Enchilada and tomatillo sauces are also usually okay if they're freshly made and don't have added sugar, but try to stay away from full-fat sour cream and full-fat cheese.

Cafeteria Chains

Cafeteria chains such as Luby's (over 1,300 in Texas) and Piccadilly (which has more than 130 cafeterias in 15 states) have a wide variety of interesting choices that make them good destinations for South Beach dieters on the go. You'll have to watch out for all the usual pitfalls, including deep-fried foods and those tempting home-baked breads and pastries, but you should easily be able to put together a good selection of healthy dishes. Cafeterias usually have extensive salad offerings, a carving station where you can get roasted chicken or turkey breast, side dishes made with fresh vegetables, and daily specials that often feature good SBD choices such as baked fish.

Event Eating

You're at a baseball game, a county fair, a street fair, the circus, or some other event. There are food booths and enticing aromas everywhere. You know the fried dough, cotton candy, and corn dogs are out. What's in? A surprisingly good number of choices.

At fairs, look for grilled chicken, shish kebab in a whole-wheat pita, salads, and vegetable wraps. You might even be able to find a slice of thin-crust veggie pizza. For a snack, try some roasted peanuts.

A ball game just isn't a ball game without a hot dog—if you want one, skip the roll, have the dog on a plate, and stick to just one. Hot dogs are high in saturated fat and often contain fillers made from refined carbohydrates, to say nothing of the chemical additives. At any arena event, like a football game or circus, there's probably a food court you can explore in addition to other food vendors. Many of these venues have finally come to realize that huge numbers of Americans are embracing healthy eating as a way of life, so you might find there are good choices to be had.

At any event, drinks are the easy part. You can always get diet soda, sugar-free lemonade or iced tea, or bottled water. On occasion, a light beer is also okay if you are not on Phase 1.

Travel Meals

Trying to find a good South Beach Diet meal while you're traveling can be a real problem. The typical airport or train terminal consists largely of assorted fast-food restaurants offering mostly burgers and pizza, interspersed with places selling candy, cinnamon buns, frozen yogurt, and other examples of poor nutrition. Today you usually need to bring your own food along on long airplane flights, which means busy travelers end up buying pre-made sandwiches simply for the convenience. On top of that, traveling is stressful—and when you're under stress, you're more vulnerable to temptation.

There are a few strategies that can help you stick to the South Beach Diet even under these circumstances. Before you start your trip, fuel up with a good meal at home. If you're not that hungry when you pass by the cookie stand, you'll be able to avoid temptation more easily. If possible, don't skip meals in order to make better time. You'll regret it later when you get ravenous and end up overeating or eating something you shouldn't. When you know you won't be able to stop for a real meal, bring along some convenient snack foods, such as low-fat string cheese. Or look for a stand selling roasted nuts—just don't buy any of the candy these stands also sell. If you're not on Phase 1 and want a sandwich, ask for whole-wheat bread and a lower-fat filling such as turkey or grilled chicken. Traveling needn't be an excuse to go off the South Beach Diet, but you may need to plan ahead to stay within the guidelines.

Ethnic Restaurants

The wonderful flavors and rich cultural heritage of ethnic cuisines make them a popular option when eating out. With a little knowledge and some flexibility, you can still easily stick to the South Beach Diet while you enjoy the world's great cooking.

American Steakhouses

A thick, juicy steak is about as American as it gets, so in a way steakhouses *are* ethnic cuisine! You can definitely eat at a steakhouse as long as you stick to the leaner beef cuts such as top sirloin or tenderloin. The weight of the steak portion is often on the menu—preferably choose a steak that is 8 ounces or less because of the saturated fat. Elsewhere on the menu, grilled pork chops, chicken, shrimp, and fish are all good alternatives. Appetizers such as green salad or shrimp cocktail are fine, but watch out for the creamy soups and deep-fried appetizers, such as fried mozzarella sticks. The side dishes at steakhouses are often heavy on potatoes in various forms, but sautéed vegetables are also on the menu. Just swap your steak fries or onion rings for some extra broccoli or sautéed spinach.

Chinese Restaurants

Worldwide, Chinese food is one of the most popular ethnic cuisines. Chinese food is often perceived as healthier than other cuisines, and in some ways it is. Authentic Chinese cooking emphasizes fresh ingredients, vegetables, seafood, and light sauces. Many dishes are stir-fried (prepared very quickly in a small amount of oil) or steamed.

Unfortunately, authentic Chinese cooking is hard to find. To accommodate the tastes of their customers, many Chinese res-

Safe Salad Dressings

South Beach dieters eat a lot of salads—they're a delicious, crunchy, filling way to get your veggies and fiber. With the right dressing, salads are also a great way to get the good fats (and extra flavor) that come with olive oil and canola oil. With the wrong dressing, however, a salad could become a source of hidden sugars and bad fats. When choosing your dressing at a restaurant, you're always safe with olive oil and vinegar. You're also likely to be okay if you stick to a small amount of regular ranch, Italian, Caesar, blue cheese, or regular vinaigrette dressing. Avoid Thousand Island, French, Russian, raspberry vinaigrette, and most fat-free dressings; they're all likely to have added sugar (more than 3 grams of sugar in 2 tablespoons)

taurants serve large portions that are heavy on meat and sauces and light on vegetables.

As with any other menu, you need to choose carefully at a Chinese restaurant. Look for healthy, lower-fat, better-carb choices such as clear soup or any combination of steamed fresh vegetables prepared with small amounts of meat, poultry, or seafood. Avoid steamed white rice, and watch out for the high-calorie, refined-carb, noodle-based entrées such as lo mein, chow fun, fried rice, and pot stickers (dumplings). Also stay away from anything on the menu that calls itself crispy or sweet-and-sour—these dishes will be deep-fried and/or have added sugar. And just as you would ask your server to take away the bread basket, ask to have the bowl of crispy noodles removed from the table. Finally, be sure to request that your food be prepared without MSG, a flavoring agent often used in Chinese cooking (and in many other prepared foods), and without cornstarch to thicken the sauce.

French Restaurants

It's hard to even know where to begin when talking about the delights of French food—be it the sophisticated cuisine of the great chefs or simple bistro fare. The good news is that French food can fit right in with the South Beach Diet because it's typically prepared with care using the freshest ingredients. When choosing a French restaurant for a meal, go for the simple Mediterranean fare typical of southern France. In this region, olive oil is the basic fat used for sautéing and salad dressings, simply prepared fish and shellfish are the most popular entrées, and fresh vegetables are the usual accompaniment. A classic French specialty, ratatouille, is made with eggplant, peppers, tomatoes, onions, and zucchini and is an ideal South Beach dish. Salade Niçoise (made with tuna) and fish Provençal (made with tomatoes and fresh herbs) are other great SBD choices.

If you're at a French restaurant featuring more elaborate fare, with dishes that have complex sauces made with butter, cream, or cheese, just make the best selections you can and ask for the sauce on the side, if possible. Your server will be able to tell you the ingredients in unfamiliar dishes and suggest substitutions. One classic dish to definitely avoid: *Canard* (duck) *à l'Orange*—

the sauce is sweetened. Ditto for *Canard aux Cerises* (cherries). Also avoid *pommes frites* (french fries) and any other potatoes. Ask for an extra serving of those delicious vegetables instead.

Of course a true French meal isn't complete without wine. By all means, have a glass of wine with your meal, preferably a red such as Beaujolais, Burgundy, or Bordeaux.

Greek and Middle Eastern Restaurants

From a South Beach Diet perspective, Greek and Middle Eastern cuisine is about as healthy as you can get. In countries such as Greece, Lebanon, Israel, and Turkey, the cooking is simple, relying heavily on fresh ingredients and olive oil for flavor. Grilled seafood, lamb, and chicken; whole grains such as bulgur and couscous; beans such as chickpeas; and fresh vegetables, fresh herbs, and feta cheese are all staples.

Some Middle Eastern classics that are fine for South Beach dieters include kibbe (grilled patties of ground lamb and bulgur), souvlaki (marinated lamb grilled on a skewer), hummus (a chickpea dip), and tzatziki (a dip made with cucumber, garlic, and yogurt). Pita bread traditionally accompanies most meals. Try asking for whole-wheat pita, or use vegetables as dippers instead.

As healthy as the food appears, there are still a few dishes to watch out for in a Greek or Middle Eastern restaurant. Pasta, rice, or potatoes are intrinsic to some favorites such as pastitsio (a sort of Greek version of lasagna) and moussaka (a casserole of eggplant, potatoes, and chopped beef or lamb). Both of these dishes also come topped with béchamel sauce, a South Beach Diet no-no since it's made with butter, flour, and whole milk. Rice is often served as a side dish; just ask for more veggies or a salad instead.

Indian Restaurants

India is a very large and very diverse country—and the cuisine is just as wide ranging. Every region has its own style of cooking, from the vegetarian dishes of the South to the lamb-based cuisine of the North, with much in between. Many Indian dishes turn out to be good South Beach Diet choices. A favorite is tandoori, in which meat, poultry, and fish are roasted at very high temperatures inside a clay oven. Other dishes to try without concern include dal (made with lentils and various other kinds of beans), curries (try chana, a chickpea curry), kachumbars (vegetable salads), raitas (salads with a tart yogurt dressing), and masala-style dishes, made with sautéed tomatoes and onions. You may also want to explore other nonmeat dishes made using spinach, eggplant, beans, or whole grains.

As in any ethnic cuisine, there are some Indian foods you should avoid. The list begins with the deep-fried appetizers such as samosas (triangular pastry filled with vegetables) and pakoras (fritters). You will also need to skip the tempting Indian breads, such as puri (puffy, deep-fried flat bread), which are very high in refined carbohydrates. Even breads like nan, which can be made with whole wheat, often have added sugar.

Also stay away from Indian dishes, such as biriyanis, in which the meat, seafood, or vegetables are cooked together with basmati rice. (You'll also have to skip basmati rice as a side dish.) Fiery vindaloos are also a problem. These stews, made with meat, poultry, or seafood, always contain potatoes. In addition, you'll need to skip the dishes made with cream, such as korma or malai.

Italian Restaurants

When you think Italian restaurant, you may think pasta—and immediately you might decide that Italian food isn't a good

Never Say Never

The beauty of the South Beach Diet is that, in the end, no food is off-limits forever. That's what makes dining out on this diet so easy and pleasurable. Once you're on Phase 3, you can occasionally enjoy foods you had to give up on Phases 1 and 2. That's because you've learned to think about food in accordance with principles of tho South Deach Dlet, and you know that you can be a little indulgent now and then because you're eating healthfully the rest of the time.

There will also be times when everyday life may intrude on your best-laid plans. When dining out with friends, family, or business associates, don't berate yourself if you slip up now and then. Keep in mind that the South Beach Diet is a lifestyle, and if you aren't happy with your choices at one meal, you can simply get back on track at the next one.

choice for a South Beach dieter. But pasta isn't a reason to forgo one of the world's great cuisines. You can easily enjoy a great Italian meal, including some pasta (if you're on Phase 2 or 3), and still stay within your South Beach Diet guidelines.

In Italy, pasta is served in small portions as a preamble to the main dish. Stick to that idea and request whole-wheat pasta with a simple tomato sauce (stay away from the creamy sauces) and a sprinkle of freshly grated Parmesan cheese. The rest of a good Italian meal is easy for South Beach dieters: salad, fresh vegetables, and grilled or roasted meat, poultry, fish, or shellfish.

There are some things to avoid in Italian restaurants, however. The bread basket tops the list, unless some good whole-grain breads can be found in it. If so, have a small piece, dipping it into extra virgin olive oil instead of slathering on the butter. Other foods to avoid are the salami and other fatty meats and cheeses in the antipasto; rice dishes (risotto); polenta (a type of cornmeal mush); and gnocchi (potato dumplings). Anything breaded and fried (fritti) is out—and that includes calamari (squid) and dishes such as veal Parmesan. Instead, order menu items that aren't battered, such as veal piccata or scaloppine.

Japanese Restaurants

In Japan, food not only tastes great, it looks great. The visual presentation of a dish is as important as its flavor. Because Japanese cooks are very concerned with capturing the essential flavor of a food, that means using only the freshest ingredients and preparing them simply, without elaborate sauces.

Many Japanese dishes are good choices for South Beach dieters. Miso soup makes a great start to a meal. Fish and shellfish are mainstays of Japanese cuisine. You'll have to skip the sushi (raw or cooked seafood or vegetables served on a platform of rice) or have just a piece or two if you're on Phase 2 or 3. You can always enjoy sashimi—slices of raw fish and shellfish served without rice. Most tofu (bean curd) dishes are a good choice, as are vegetable dishes such as edamame (soybeans).

A favorite way to enjoy grilled dishes the Japanese way is teppanyaki style—the food is cooked right in front of you on a very hot grill. Teriyaki-style dishes are also grilled, but the marinade is sweet and contains added sugar—so avoid them. Also stay away from tempura dishes, which are battered and deep-fried. Another Japanese favorite that's a good choice is shabu-shabu, a fondue-style dish where you cook slices of meat and vegetables in broth at your table.

Noodles and rice are the primary starches in Japanese cooking. Most noodles are made from refined grains such as wheat and rice. However, soba noodles (which are made from buckwheat) can be tried in moderation if you're on Phase 2 or 3. Avoid the refined carbs of the white rice by asking for brown rice instead.

Korean Restaurants

One of the lesser-known cuisines, Korean food is a complex and delicious blend of many different culinary influences. Because Korea is a peninsula, the cooking includes many fish and seafood dishes—good choices for your South Beach diet.

A favorite Korean cooking style is bulgogi, or barbecue. Thin slices of beef, poultry, pork, fish, or shellfish are marinated in a fragrant barbecue sauce and then grilled tableside—in many restaurants, you can grill your own. The grilled pieces are wrapped in lettuce leaves before eating. Because the barbecue marinade is typically made with a small amount of sugar or honey and much of it burns off during grilling, you can enjoy this unusual meal without worry—just don't add any additional sauce. Small dishes of pickled vegetables (kimchee) and other small plates of the chef's choosing accompany the meal.

As with all Asian cuisines, noodles and rice are an important part of Korean meals. Skip the noodle dishes, though you could try a small portion of those made with buckwheat noodles, if you're on Phase 2 or beyond. You should be able to get brown rice instead of white as an accompaniment to a meal, but avoid dishes with *bap* in the name—these are made with white rice. Bimibap, a rice casserole made with pieces of meat, vegetables, and eggs, is a very popular Korean dish—if you're on Phase 3, it's okay to have a taste if someone else orders it.

Mexican Restaurants

Tacos, tortillas, quesadillas, and burritos aren't the only dishes in Mexican cuisine. True Mexican cooking, as opposed to the fast-food version, is full of complex and subtle flavors and has great regional variation. While the basic starches of Mexican cooking—tortillas, rice, and corn in many forms—are high in refined carbs and should be eaten only in limited amounts (and never on Phase 1), there's still plenty on the menu you can enjoy. Look especially for grilled items such as pollo asado (grilled chicken) and seafood dishes. Enjoy salads and interesting vegetables such as jicama (a crunchy root vegetable) as side dishes, along with fresh salsa. If you're on Phase 2, it's okay to have a whole-wheat tortilla along with your meal—but stick to just one. And stay away from the deep-fried tortilla chips.

Thai Restaurants

Thai cuisine is growing in popularity, and with good reason. The interesting and sometimes fiery flavor blends of Thai cooking are unusual and delicious. Unfortunately, the favorite menu item in Thai restaurants is pad thai, a classic noodle dish made with rice noodles, shrimp, scallions, eggs, pressed bean curd, bean sprouts, and chopped peanuts, all in a slightly sweet sauce. Most other Thai dishes are also based on noodles or rice, and many of the sauces include some added sugar, so you'll have to be careful. Watch out for anything with coconut milk (regular coconut milk has a lot of saturated fat, and restaurants do not typically use the "light" version), sweet-and-sour sauce, oyster sauce, brown sauce, or garlic sauce. Fish sauce, or nam pla, is the Thai equivalent of soy sauce and is acceptable.

Your best choices are anything that is stir-fried, sautéed, or steamed with herbs such as Thai basil or lemon grass. In the salad part of the menu, look for Thai specialties such as grilled beef salad or a small green papaya salad (if you're on Phase 2 or 3). Among the entrées, choose dishes that are stir-fried with vegetables, such as chicken pad prik king (chicken with Thai basil, string beans, chile paste, and lime leaves). When ordering stir-fries, ask to have the ingredients stir-fried in broth rather than in garlic or brown sauce. Grilled chicken or beef satés, which come with peanut sauce, are good as well. Among the curry dishes, look for those that do not contain coconut milk, such as country style.

Vietnamese Restaurants

The cuisine of Vietnam is mildly spicy and quite varied. The influences of China, Thailand, India, and France can all be detected in the intriguing dishes of this small country. The primary flavorings are nuoc nam, or fish sauce, and nuoc cham, a spicy dipping sauce made with fish sauce, lime juice, sugar, garlic, and chiles. (Because nuoc cham contains sugar, use only small amounts.) Saté, a paste of peanuts, garlic, and chiles, is often added to stir-fried dishes.

Mild curries are popular in Vietnamese cooking; and the flavors of mint, lemon grass, coriander, ginger, and star anise pervade many dishes. Fresh herbs (or rau thom) are served with just about every meal, along with table salad (or rau song), made with lettuce, cucumbers, bean sprouts, shredded carrots, and other vegetables.

When ordering, you'll have to avoid spring rolls, summer rolls, dumplings, the famous Vietnamese beef noodle soup called pho bo, and all the other dishes that use rice noodles and other noodles. That still leaves some good options. Appetizers featuring ingredients such as beef or seafood wrapped in lettuce leaves are one possibility. Also check the menu for salad selections, which often use delicious ingredients such as green papaya and tamarind in the dressings. You're also well off with grilled, stir-fried, and steamed dishes, shrimp and other seafood, and vegetarian combinations using bean curd.

Enjoy Yourself

Dining out often while sticking to the South Beach Diet may take a bit of adjusting, but if you follow the strategies suggested here, you'll find that you can happily eat just about anywhere, no matter what phase of the diet you're on. The following pages give you many good menu choices in more than 100 restaurants. Whether you're out for fast food or an evening of fine dining, whether you're on Phase 1 or Phase 3, there is always something good for you to eat. You won't feel deprived because you will still be able to eat most of your favorite foods—but in healthier and often more flavorful ways. Moreover, with every meal you order, you'll know you're taking positive steps toward losing weight and improving your health the South Beach Diet way.

CHAIN AND FAMILY
RESTAURANTS

It's almost inevitable that anyone, even a South Beach dieter, will eat at a chain restaurant sometime. But if you're armed with the information in this guide, you won't have to go it alone. To help you deal with the fast-food dilemma, we've selected more than 75 chains (including some upscale family restaurants) that offer dishes that fit in with the South Beach Diet guidelines. The restaurants included are all familiar names, many with hundreds of franchises.

For each restaurant, we suggest some Best Choices and often provide suggestions for making a particular dish healthier. To further assist you, we've included a nutritional analysis for the diet-friendly menu items and have assigned the diet phase that applies. This nutritional data has been provided by the restaurants and is as current as possible. Where no analyses were available, we have still made menu recommendations based on the principles of the diet.

Unless otherwise indicated, a nutritional analysis reflects everything that is part of a dish. For example, we tell you whether a burger is analyzed with or without the bun, a Caesar salad with or without croutons. Simply removing refined carbs can often take a dish from Phase 3 to Phase 1, and we have assigned the phases accordingly. We have also researched ingredients and cooking methods to find out how a dish is prepared. For example, if a restaurant cooks its vegetables in butter, it's reflected in the phase recommendation. That's why broccoli, which looks like it should be a "1," could be labeled a "3." South Beach dieters need to be vigilant when it comes to evaluating the menu items in fast-casual restaurants, especially if you're on Phase 1. Ask your server to help steer you to the healthiest choices.

~~~ Applebee's Neighborhood ~~~ Grill & Bar

More than 1,600 locations in 49 states
(913) 967-4000, www.applebees.com

NOTE: Applebee's makes nutritional information available for only some of its dishes. We have, however, listed a few other choices that fit in with the South Beach Diet nutritional principles. Because we do not have specific data for these dishes, talk to your server if you have questions about the ingredients in a dish, and be especially vigilant if you are on Phase 1.

Applebee's takes the neighborhood concept seriously: The décor of each restaurant reflects its locale, with photographs and memorabilia highlighting area history and notable figures. In addition to the regular menu items, Applebee's offers specially prepared dishes that would, at first glance, seem to be legitimate on the South Beach Diet. The Grilled Tilapia with Mango Salsa, for instance, comes on a bed of rice pilaf. It's easy to make this into an excellent South Beach Diet choice, however—just ask for vegetables instead of the rice and hold the fruit salsa if you're on Phase 1.

BEST CHOICES

The regular menu at Applebee's has some good South Beach Diet–friendly options. Check out the grill items, such as the Applebee's House Sirloin or Sizzling Chicken Skillet. Ask your server for additional veggies instead of the rice or garlic mashed potatoes that accompany almost all grill items. Most of Applebee's main-course salads are another good option—try the Grilled Shrimp Skewer Salad with Lemon Herb Vinaigrette Dressing.

RECOMMENDED DISHES

SANDWICHES

Menu Item	Calories	Fat (g)	Sat. Fat (g)	Carbs (g)	Fiber (g)	Phase
Tango Chicken Sandwich	370	9	n/a	38	8	3

GRILL MENU

Menu Item	Calories	Fat (g)	Sat. Fat (g)	Carbs (g)	Fiber (g)	Phase
Applebee's House Sirloin	n/a	n/a	n/a	n/a	n/a	1
Bourbon Street Steak	n/a	n/a	n/a	n/a	n/a	1
Grilled Tilapia with Mango Salsa (with pilaf)*	320	6	n/a	27	9	2
Sizzling Chicken Skillet	360	4	n/a	43	10	2

*Nutritional analysis includes pilaf. Eliminating the pilaf reduces carbohydrates and calories in this dish.

SALADS

Menu Item	Calories	Fat (g)	Sat. Fat (g)	Carbs (g)	Fiber (g)	Phase
Grilled Italian Chicken Caesar Salad (no croutons)	n/a	n/a	n/a	n/a	n/a	1
Grilled Shrimp Skewer Salad (with dressing)	210	2	n/a	22	7	1
Mesquite Chicken Salad (with dressing)	250	4	n/a	42	7	3

—∾— Arby's —∾—

More than 3,400 locations worldwide
(800) 487-2729, www.arbys.com

Arby's gets its name from the initials for roast beef, right? Wrong! The corporate name actually comes from the Raffel brothers—Forrest and Leroy, the two siblings who founded the chain in 1964. Today Arby's is still best known for its roast beef sandwiches, but the menu also includes a wide variety of other sandwiches, in fact, the emphasis on sandwiches makes finding a good South Beach Diet choice at Arby's a little challenging. You can avoid the bad carbs from the white flour of the sandwich bread simply by not eating it, but there are only a few acceptable fillings. None of the side dishes, such as potato cakes, curly fries, or onion petals, are good choices. Fortunately, Arby's now offers some acceptable salads and wraps.

BEST CHOICES

Among the classic roast beef sandwiches, those that contain moderate amounts of only roast beef are fine—if you skip the sesame seed bun or eat only a small part of it. The Regular Roast Beef Sandwich is a reasonable choice. Even better would be the Junior Roast Beef Sandwich. In both cases, toss half or all of the sesame seed bun. The best salad is the Martha's Vineyard, with mixed greens, grilled chicken, diced apples, dried cranberries, grape tomatoes, and shredded cheddar cheese—with added sliced almonds. Don't use the raspberry vinaigrette the salad is served with; ask for oil and vinegar instead.

RECOMMENDED DISHES

SANDWICHES

Menu Item	Calories	Fat (g)	Sat. Fat (g)	Carbs (g)	Fiber (g)	Phase
Junior Roast Beef Sandwich	270	9	4	34	2	3
Regular Roast Beef Sandwich	320	13	6	34	2	3
Sourdough Roast Beef Melt	300	12	4.5	31	1	3

SALADS

Menu Item	Calories	Fat (g)	Sat. Fat (g)	Carbs (g)	Fiber (g)	Phase
Martha's Vineyard (with almonds, no dressing)	330	15	4.5	25	5	2
Santa Fe (no dressing)	520	29	9	40	5	3

—⚬— Au Bon Pain —⚬—

More than 230 cafés nationwide
(800) 825-5227, www.aubonpain.com

Au Bon Pain began as a bakery in 1978, based at Boston's historic Faneuil Hall Marketplace. Today the chain still offers fresh-baked bread at its cafés—along with a variety of salads, soups, stews, sandwiches, and wraps. Au Bon Pain can be a good lunch destination, especially if you're on Phase 2 and beyond.

BEST CHOICES

Soups, stews, and salads are the best choices at Au Bon Pain, with quite a variety in reasonably sized portions. A serving of soup or stew makes a good start to a satisfying lunch, and it can also be an excellent snack. At Au Bon Pain, the menu typically offers two different stews and four different soups, so on any given day, you should be able to find at least one good choice. Look for the soups that have the most vegetables and the fewest starches—Southwest Vegetable Soup is a good option. If one of the soups doesn't appeal to you, have a salad. The choices at Au Bon Pain are wide-ranging and go beyond the usual fast-food standards. Keep in mind that if you order a Caesar Salad, and it comes with croutons, that makes it a Phase 3 dish. Skipping the croutons makes it Phase 1.

The sandwiches are a bit more of a challenge for a South Beach dieter. But because many of the breads at Au Bon Pain are made from whole grains, they're acceptable.

You can also create your own sandwich from either smoked turkey breast, Black Forest ham, roast beef, tuna, or grilled chicken breast with your choice of bread and toppings. If you choose turkey, tuna, or grilled chicken on a multigrain bread and limit the toppings to the vegetable choices (romaine lettuce, alfalfa sprouts, and the like), it's possible to put together a South Beach Diet meal. In fact, eating only half of any of these sandwiches is your best bet. Ditto for the wraps (which come on lavash) and the baked sandwiches (which come on focaccia). Stay away from any sandwiches on breads made with refined white flour, such as baguettes, croissants, white bread, or white rolls—and skip the baguette slice that comes with the salads.

RECOMMENDED DISHES

SOUPS AND STEWS

Menu Item	Calories	Fat (g)	Sat. Fat (g)	Carbs (g)	Fiber (g)	Phase
French Moroccan Tomato Lentil Soup (1½ cups)	165	2	2	29	9	1
Garden Vegetable Soup (1½ cups)	60	2	0	10	3	3
Jamaican Black Bean Soup (1½ cups)	165	1	0	40	21	3
Southwest Vegetable Soup (1½ cups)	255	5	1	35	6	3
Tomato Florentine Soup (1½ cups)	105	3	1	15	2	1
Tuscan Vegetable Soup (1 cup)	130	3	1.5	20	3	3
Vegetable Beef Barley Soup (1 cup)	80	2	1	11	2	2
Chicken Chili (1½ cups)	315	7	1.5	42	7	1
Mediterranean Seafood Stew (1 cup)	140	4	1	12	1	3

SALADS

Menu Item	Calories	Fat (g)	Sat. Fat (g)	Carbs (g)	Fiber (g)	Phase
Caesar (with croutons)*	240	11	6	23	4	3
Chicken Caesar (with croutons)*	530	22	10	40	4	3
Chicken Pesto	420	30	8	14	5	1
Mediterranean Chicken*	290	16	4	14	5	1
Thai Chicken*	140	3	0.5	14	6	1
Tuna Garden*	400	24	3.5	25	6	1
Tuna Niçoise*	300	15	2.5	19	5	3

*Nutritional analysis includes dressing. Eliminating the dressing reduces carbohydrates, fat, and calories in this dish.

SANDWICHES AND WRAPS

Menu Item	Calories	Fat (g)	Sat. Fat (g)	Carbs (g)	Fiber (g)	Phase
Roasted Portobello, Goat Cheese Sandwich*	560	27	8	63	6	3
Chicken Salsa Wrap*	440	8	1.5	68	8	3
Chicken Caesar Wrap*	591	24	8	63	5	3
Fields and Feta Wrap*	551	10	4	90	14	3
Mediterranean Wrap*	571	22	2.5	80	9	3
Southwest Tuna Wrap*	541	25	7	68	7	3

*Nutritional analysis is based on the chain's suggested bread. Choose multigrain bread instead for a Phase 2 sandwich.

—✺— Back Yard Burgers —✺—

More than 150 restaurants in 18 states
(901) 367-0888, www.backyardburgers.com

Back Yard Burgers is a relatively new entry in the fast-food burger market. The first restaurant opened in 1987 in Missouri, and the chain has expanded since then to 18 states, mostly in the Southeast and Midwest. Although the chain began with drive-thrus, today almost all Back Yard Burger restaurants feature a full dining room.

BEST CHOICES

Back Yard Burgers offers slightly more good options for the South Beach dieter than most chains. While there are over 10 burgers on the menu, the only one we recommend is the Back Yard Burger Jr., which is smaller and lower in saturated fat. Eat it without the bun. The signature chicken sandwiches are made with skinless, boneless breasts that are charbroiled. The Savory Chicken Sandwich and Blackened Chicken Sandwich are both good, as long as you toss the bread. Avoid the Honey Mustard and Hawaiian versions. The Garden Veggie Sandwich is a possibility; again, toss the bread and skip the ketchup. In the salad department, Back Yard Burgers offers two chicken options that are excellent choices: Blackened Chicken and Charbroiled Chicken. Choose SBD-friendly salad dressings, such as ranch or Italian.

RECOMMENDED DISHES

SANDWICHES

Menu Item	Calories	Fat (g)	Sat. Fat (g)	Carbs (g)	Fiber(g)	Phase
Back Yard Burger Jr. (with bun)*	310	17	6	38	2	3
Savory Chicken Sandwich*	230	6	2	36	1	3
Blackened Chicken Sandwich*	290	11	3	39	2	3
Garden Veggie Sandwich*	240	6	1.5	47	6	3

*Nutritional analysis includes bread. Eliminating the bread reduces carbohydrates, fat, and calories in this dish.

SALADS (no dressing)

Menu Item	Calories	Fat (g)	Sat. Fat	Carbs (g)	Fiber (g)	Phase
Blackened Chicken Salad	160	4	1.5	11	3	1
Charbroiled Chicken Salad	140	3	1	11	3	1
Garden Fresh Side Salad	25	0	0	5	1	1

—⚬— Baja Fresh Mexican Grill —⚬—

More than 400 locations in 23 states
(877) 225-2373, www.bajafresh.com

Restaurants in the Baja Fresh chain feature contemporary décor, salsa bars, and exhibition kitchens that let you watch the food being prepared in full view. Since the chain was founded in 1990, the restaurants have emphasized Mexican dishes made using only the freshest ingredients—the numerous different salsas are all prepared fresh daily.

Mexican food is always a challenge for South Beach dieters. In addition to the bottomless supply of tortilla chips, all too many dishes contain refined carbs in the form of flour tortillas and rice. Fortunately, the menu at Baja Fresh still has some good options—you can even have a burrito.

BEST CHOICES

The Bare Burrito and the Veggie and Cheese Bare Burrito are a great way to enjoy burrito flavor without the refined carbs. Served in a bowl, they contain all the ingredients for the burrito filling, minus the flour tortilla. The Bare Burrito features charbroiled chicken, grilled peppers, chiles and onions, rice, black or pinto beans, pico de gallo, and salsa verde. The Veggie and Cheese Bare Burrito contains grilled peppers, chiles and onions, rice, black or pinto beans, lettuce, Jack cheese, sour cream, pico de gallo, and Salsa Baja. Holding the rice can make these Phase 3 dishes suitable for Phase 1. The beans are fine in any phase.

continued

Some of the salads at Baja Fresh are good choices if you're on Phase 3. Try the Chile Lime Chicken Salad, featuring warm chicken tenders topped with cheese, black beans, roasted corn, roasted peppers, and tomatoes. Ask for the Sweet Tomato Chutney on the side, and skip the tortilla chips. Baja Ensalada—a sort of Mexican Caesar salad—with charbroiled steak, chicken, or shrimp is another good choice. Here, too, eliminating the toppings and chips can make these Phase 1. Whatever phase you're on, your best choices at Baja are the charbroiled steak, chicken, or fish. Add a Side Salad with Salsa Verde.

RECOMMENDED DISHES

BURRITOS

Menu Item	Calories	Fat (g)	Sat. Fat (g)	Carbs (g)	Fiber (g)	Phase
Bare Burrito (chicken)*	650	7	1.5	99	22	3
Veggie and Cheese Bare Burrito*	590	10	4	102	21	3

*Nutritional analysis includes rice. Eliminating the rice reduces carbohydrates and calories in this dish.

SALADS (no dressing)

Menu Item	Calories	Fat (g)	Sat. Fat (g)	Carbs (g)	Fiber (g)	Phase
Baja Ensalada (chicken)	310	7	2	18	7	3
Baja Ensalada (shrimp)	230	6	2	18	6	3
Baja Ensalada (steak)	450	18	7	18	6	3
Mahi Mahi Ensalada	310	12	3	22	10	3
Chile Lime Chicken Salad*	510	15	3	50	11	3
Side Salad with Salsa Verde	85	3	1	13	4	3

*Nutritional analysis includes toppings, chutney, and tortilla chips. Eliminating these reduces carbohydrates, fat, and calories in this dish.

CHARBROILED ENTRÉES

Menu Item	Calories	Fat (g)	Sat. Fat (g)	Carbs (g)	Fiber (g)	Phase
Charbroiled Steak (5 oz)	318	14	6	0	0	1
Charbroiled Chicken (6 oz)	224	3.5	0.5	0	0	1
Charbroiled Fish (6 oz)	207	3	1	1	0	1

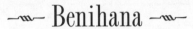

—⚒— Benihana —⚒—

Nearly 100 restaurants nationwide
(800) 327-3369, www.benihana.com

As much entertainment as fine dining, Benihana restaurants feature teppanyaki-style cooking—dishes prepared tableside on a steel grill called a hibachi. The dazzling knifework and other effects by the highly trained chefs who do the grilling are part of the experience. The Benihana approach dates back to 1964, when the flamboyant founder, Rocky Aoki, opened his first restaurant in New York City. The combination of showmanship and good food brought him a lot of attention and introduced Japanese cooking to the United States.

BEST CHOICES

Teppanyaki cooking features beef, chicken, shrimp, fish, and vegetables, all sliced, diced, and cooked on the grill right in front of you. All these dishes are good South Beach Diet choices. With all the grilled dishes, the only thing you have to be careful of is the white rice that accompanies your meal. Ask for more vegetables instead. The Benihana Vegetable Delight comes with Japanese noodles. Have the chef eliminate them unless you're on Phase 3.

continued

RECOMMENDED DISHES

ENTRÉES

Menu Item	Calories	Fat (g)	Sat. Fat (g)	Carbs (g)	Fiber (g)	Phase
Benihana Vegetable Delight*	140	5	0	22	6	3
Benihana Shrimp (6 oz)	230	8	1	3	0	1
Hibachi Chicken (7 oz)	400	21	9	4	1	1
Benihana Chicken (5 oz)	220	7	1	2	0	1
Hibachi Steak (7 oz)	360	18	5	2	0	1
Benihana Special Steak and Lobster (5 oz each)	450	20	5	5	1	1
Benihana Rocky's Choice (5 oz steak)	270	14	4	2	0	1
Benihana Rocky's Choice (3 oz chicken)	150	4.5	1	7	2	1
Benihana Steak (5 oz)	260	15	4.5	4	0	1

*Nutritional analysis includes noodles. Eliminating the noodles reduces the carbohydrates, fat, and calories in this dish.

—⚬— Bennigan's Grill & Tavern —⚬—

More than 275 restaurants in 33 states
(800) 727-8355, www.bennigans.com

NOTE: Nutritional information was not available for this establishment. However, we have provided some Best Choices that fit in with the South Beach Diet nutritional principles. Because we do not have specific data for these dishes, talk to your server if you have questions about the ingredients in a dish, and be especially vigilant if you are on Phase 1.

The relaxed, upbeat atmosphere at Bennigan's Grill & Tavern makes this a favorite for family dining. Bennigan's is famed for hamburgers, but recent menu changes have added variety to the entrées—and made them more South Beach Diet friendly.

BEST CHOICES

The new menu at Bennigan's has some interesting main-course salads, such as the Greek Chicken Salad and Cajun-Grilled Salmon Caesar Salad. (Just stay away from the smoky honey Dijon dressing.) New entrées such as Mediterranean Grilled Chicken (without the garlic mashed potatoes) and Grilled Atlantic Salmon are good choices. If you can't decide, try the mix and match entrée option, which lets you combine any two items on a list that includes Fire-Grilled Top Sirloin, Cajun Shrimp Skewer, Southwest Grilled Chicken Breast, and Cajun Salmon. The side dishes at Bennigan's are more varied than in a lot of similar restaurants. Look for black beans, broccoli, green beans, and roasted vegetables as substitutes for potatoes and rice. The appetizers at Bennigan's are unfortunately all off the South Beach Diet radar—just about every one is breaded and deep-fried and unacceptably high in saturated fat.

—⚬— Blimpie —⚬—

More than 1,600 restaurants nationwide and 13 countries
(800) 477-6256, www.blimpie.com

There was a time, back in the early '60s, when submarine sandwiches were a daring new idea. The concept of a sub shop appealed to three young guys who had been high school buddies, and in 1964 they opened the first Blimpie restaurant in Hoboken, New Jersey. Prices for their generous sandwiches ranged from 35 cents all the way up to 95 cents. The first store was very successful right from the start, and over the years the partners expanded their business into the large chain it is today. Overstuffed sandwiches remain the Blimpie trademark.

BEST CHOICES

Blimpie has been reasonably responsive to consumer demand for choices that don't include a lot of refined carbs. The menu offers a good number of salads for a sandwich chain. Try the Chef Salad, Tuna Salad, or Seafood Salad. Skip the salads that come in tortilla bowls. You can also create your own SBD-friendly salad, choosing from the ham, roast beef, turkey breast, or tuna available for the sandwiches. Avoid the high fat content of the other cold cuts. Most of the available dressings are fine, but stay away from the low-fat, honey mustard, and cheese-based choices.

As far as sandwiches go, we prefer that you eat the low-fat filling without the bread because no 100 percent whole-wheat breads or wraps are currently available. Check with your server to be sure.

RECOMMENDED DISHES

SOUPS AND SALADS

Menu Item	Calories	Fat (g)	Sat. Fat (g)	Carbs (g)	Fiber (g)	Phase
Garden Vegetable Soup (8 oz)	80	0.5	0	14	3	**3**
Vegetable Beef Soup (8 oz)	80	1.5	0.5	13	2	1
Chef Salad*	210	9	4.5	9	3	1
Seafood Salad*	120	5	0.5	15	3	1
Tuna Salad*	260	19	2.5	8	3	1

*Nutritional analysis includes dressing. Eliminating the dressing reduces carbohydrates, fat, and calories in this dish.

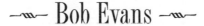

Bob Evans

More than 580 restaurants in 20 states
(800) 272-7675, www.bobevans.com

Friendly service and quality home-style food at a fair price are the distinguishing features at Bob Evans restaurants. The average check isn't much higher than for a fast-food hamburger meal—and the selection for South Beach dieters is much better. This chain, located mostly in the Midwest and Atlantic states, began in Ohio in 1953. Bob Evans was a farmer who also ran a small roadside restaurant; truckers spread the word about his homemade sausage, and the chain grew from there. The company stays in touch with its country roots by maintaining the Bob Evans Farm in Rio Grande, Ohio, a national tourist destination featuring the original Bob Evans Restaurant; the Homestead, now on the National Register of Historic Places; and special events, including the Bob Evans Farm Festival.

BEST CHOICES

South Beach dieters will find not just one but two acceptable fish dishes on the menu: Grilled Catfish and Grilled Salmon Fillet; there's also a nice, plain Grilled Chicken. We have labeled the salmon and chicken as Phase 3 because they come topped with a large deep-fried onion ring. Skipping that onion ring makes both of these dishes Phase 1. For the two sides, choose from the Broccoli Florets, Green Beans with Ham, or Garden Side Salad (no croutons). The slow-roasted Pork Loin, available only on the dinner menu, is another good choice (substitute extra broccoli for the mashed potatoes).

RECOMMENDED DISHES

ENTRÉES

Menu Item	Calories	Fat (g)	Sat. Fat (g)	Carbs (g)	Fiber (g)	Phase
Grilled New Orleans Catfish (1 piece)	270	18	4	4	2	1
Salmon Fillet (plain)*	402	20	4	12	1	3
Grilled Chicken (1 piece, plain)*	359	20	2	12	1	3
Pork Loin (1 piece)	117	6	2	4	0	1

*Nutritional analysis includes deep-fried onion ring. Eliminating it reduces carbohydrates, fat, and calories in this dish.

SIDE DISHES

Menu Item	Calories	Fat (g)	Sat. Fat (g)	Carbs (g)	Fiber (g)	Phase
Broccoli Florets	44	1	0	8	5	1
Green Beans with Ham	51	2	1	5	2	1
Garden Side Salad (no croutons)	23	0	0	5	2	1

—∿— Bonefish Grill —∿—

More than 75 restaurants in 17 states
(866) 880-2226, www.bonefishgrill.com

NOTE: Nutritional information was not available for this establishment. However, we have provided some Best Choices that fit in with the South Beach Diet nutritional principles. Because we do not have specific data for these dishes, talk to your server if you have questions about the ingredients in a dish, and be especially vigilant if you are on Phase 1.

A polished casual chain of seafood restaurants, Bonefish Grill specializes in fresh fish prepared over an oak-burning fire. The daily menu features a variety of eight or more fresh fish choices, as well as a broad array of original sauces and toppings diners can pair with the fish of their choice. The fish offerings, combined with the sleek interior and attentive service, make this chain practically designed for South Beach dieters.

BEST CHOICES

On any given day, diners at Bonefish Grill can usually choose from rainbow trout, Atlantic salmon, mahi mahi, Gulf grouper, Chilean sea bass, ahi tuna, and Atlantic swordfish. Seasonal offerings include Antarctic butterfish, monkfish, and Caribbean snapper. Top any of these grilled fish choices with an acceptable sauce, such as Bellaire (artichoke hearts, sun-dried tomatoes, goat cheese, and lemon basil) or Walker's Wood (mushrooms and sun-dried tomatoes).

If you'd rather not have fish, Bonefish Grill offers some other good SBD-friendly options, such as Chicken Marsala, Sirloin Steak, and Lily's Chicken (roasted with goat cheese, wilted spinach, artichokes, and lemon basil sauce).

Acceptable appetizers include Saucy Shrimp (in a lime tomato garlic sauce with feta cheese), Mussels Josephine (sautéed with tomatoes and garlic), and Ahi Tuna Sashimi. All the salads, such as the Florida Cobb Salad, are acceptable (just ask them to hold the bacon). The side dishes are limited—your only option here is the Steamed Vegetable Medley.

—◆— Boston Market —◆—

More than 630 restaurants in 28 states
(800) 365-7000, www.bostonmarket.com

Don't feel like cooking tonight? Stop by Boston Market and pick up a full meal to take home for the family. Boston Market, now a wholly owned subsidiary of McDonald's Corporation, practically invented the home-meal replacement concept. The fairly wide range of entrées, plus vegetable choices that are a little more interesting than typical fast-food fare, make this chain a good take-out or eat-in place for those on the South Beach diet.

BEST CHOICES

Among the entrées, the variations on Rotisserie Chicken white meat quarters are all SBD-friendly, especially if you choose the skinless and wingless versions. The Rotisserie Turkey is another good choice. Round out your entrée with some of the hot side dishes, such as the Green Beans, Steamed Vegetable Medley, or Butternut Squash. If you'd prefer a salad entrée, go for the plain Caesar Salad or Rotisserie Chicken Caesar Salad (eliminating the croutons from a main course Caesar takes it from a Phase 3 to a Phase 1 dish). The Asian Rotisserie Chicken Salad is another good option (hold the toasted noodles and go easy on the dressing). For all the salads, skip the corn bread.

RECOMMENDED DISHES

ENTRÉES

Menu Item	Calories	Fat (g)	Sat. Fat (g)	Carbs (g)	Fiber (g)	Phase
Garlic Rotisserie Chicken (white, no skin/wing)	170	4	1	2	0	1
Spicy Tuscan Rotisserie Chicken (white)	200	5	1	4	0	1
Rotisserie Turkey	170	1	0	3	0	1

SOUPS AND SALADS

Menu Item	Calories	Fat (g)	Sat. Fat (g)	Carbs (g)	Fiber (g)	Phase
Tortilla Soup (no toppings)	80	4.5	1	7	1	1
Hearty Chicken Noodle Soup	100	4.5	1.5	8	0	3
Asian Rotisserie Chicken Salad (no noodles or dressing)	270	5	1.5	22	7	2
Caesar Side Salad*	300	26	4.5	13	1	3
Caesar Salad Entrée*	470	40	9	17	3	3
Rotisserie Chicken Caesar Salad*	640	44	11	19	3	3

*Nutritional analysis includes croutons. Eliminating the croutons reduces carbohydrates, fat, and calories in this dish.

SIDE DISHES

Menu Item	Calories	Fat (g)	Sat. Fat (g)	Carbs (g)	Fiber (g)	Phase
Butternut Squash	150	6	4	25	6	2
Green Beans	70	4	0.5	6	2	1
Steamed Vegetable Medley	30	0	0	6	2	2

⟋⟍ Bubba Gump Shrimp Co. ⟋⟍

15 locations nationwide
(877) SAY GUMP, www.bubbagump.com

NOTE: Nutritional information was not available for this establishment. However, we have provided some Best Choices that fit in with the South Beach Diet nutritional principles. Because we do not have specific data for these dishes, talk to your server if you have questions about the ingredients in a dish, and be especially vigilant if you are on Phase 1.

Bubba Gump Shrimp Co. restaurants began in 1996 as a joint venture with Paramount Pictures—the theme is based on the hit movie *Forrest Gump.* These destination restaurants are all at waterfront locations and feature casual dining with décor from the film. Needless to say, the menu is heavy on shrimp and other seafood.

BEST CHOICES

As long as they're prepared in acceptable ways, fish and shellfish are excellent choices for South Beach dieters. Acceptable means grilled, broiled, baked, sautéed, or steamed—but never breaded or battered and deep-fried. At Bubba Gump Shrimp Co., shrimp and other seafood are prepared in all of these ways. Read the menu carefully, and avoid anything that's labeled as breaded, deep-fried, popcorn, or ping pong. The seafood choices you're left with are reasonably good—variations on Steamed Shrimp, Cajun Shrimp Caesar Salad (without croutons), and Charbroiled Cajun Mahi Mahi. If you're not a seafood fan, consider the Chicken Cobb Salad (hold the bacon) or Steak New Orleans. The problem at Bubba Gump Shrimp Co. is the side dishes. The choices are very limited: mashed potatoes, french fries, rice, and coleslaw. Ask your server for a house or Caesar salad instead.

–ᴡᴡ– Burger King –ᴡᴡ–

More than 11,000 restaurants worldwide
(305) 378-3535, www.bk.com

Once you take away the burger, the french fries, the chicken nuggets, and the milkshakes at a fast-food burger place, what's left? Surprisingly, at Burger King you can make some fairly good selections and enjoy a reasonable meal. You can even have the occasional burger—Burger King now offers bunless burgers on a plate—and order a side salad instead of fries. As a conscientious South Beach dieter, skip the ketchup, hold the cheese, and watch out for fat-free salad dressings that contain added sugar.

BEST CHOICES

To go bunless at Burger King, ask your server, because the option isn't prominent on the menu. Ditto for the side salad instead of fries. Your best beef burger choices are the plain Hamburger, followed by the Angus Burger, and then the Whopper. Even without the bun, these are assigned Phase 3 because of our concern about saturated fat. Better yet is the BK VEGGIE Burger without the bun. Many of these burgers come with lettuce and tomato and optional fire-grilled onions, which are all fine (always hold the sugar-laden ketchup!). But your best bet of all is the signature TENDERGRILL Chicken, which is fine for a Phase 1 dieter (without the bun and honey mustard).

Burger King also now offers four meal-sized fire-grilled salads that are good alternatives to burgers: Chicken Caesar Salad, Shrimp Caesar Salad, Chicken Garden Salad, and Shrimp Garden Salad. Hold the croutons on all. The garlic Caesar dressing and garden ranch dressings are fine, but don't fall for the fat-free honey mustard dressing—it has added sugar.

continued

47

BURGERS AND SANDWICHES

Menu Item	Calories	Fat (g)	Sat. Fat (g)	Carbs (g)	Fiber (g)	Phase
Hamburger (no bun)	140	10	4.5	0	1	3
Angus Steak Burger (no bun)	260	18	7	0	0	3
Whopper (letttuce and tomato, no bun)	250	20	9	2	0	3
BK VEGGIE Burger (no bun)	255	13.5	3	16	6	1
TENDERGRILL Chicken Sandwich (lettuce and tomato, no bun, no honey mustard)	160	4	1	3	1	1

TENDERGRILL AND TENDERCRISP SALADS (no dressing, no croutons)

Menu Item	Calories	Fat (g)	Sat. Fat (g)	Carbs (g)	Fiber (g)	Phase
Chicken Caesar Salad	190	7	3	9	1	1
Chicken Garden Salad	210	7	3	12	2	1
Shrimp Caesar Salad	180	10	3	9	2	1
Shrimp Garden Salad	200	10	3	12	3	1
Side Garden Salad	20	0	0	4	1	1

—⚓— Captain D's —⚓—

Nearly 600 restaurants in 23 states
(800) 550-4877, www.captainds.com

When you think of quick-service restaurants, you almost always think of hamburgers and fries—seafood doesn't immediately come to mind. At Captain D's, however, high–quality seafood served fast is the goal, and hamburgers aren't even on the menu (though french fries are).

BEST CHOICES

Fish is a mainstay of the South Beach Diet, but only if it's broiled, baked, or poached—never breaded or battered and fried. As at any quick-serve restaurant, many of the fish dishes at Captain D's are indeed fried and shouldn't be ordered. Ditto for many of the side dishes, such as hushpuppies. Fortunately, at this chain some of the fish and shrimp dishes on the menu can be ordered broiled or baked instead of fried, which expands the SBD-friendly options considerably.

The best choices are the three–piece Baked Fish Dinner and the Baked Salmon Dinner. Your server will be happy to replace the rice pilaf with an additional serving of Broccoli, Green Beans, Tuscan Vegetables, or a side salad. Doing so takes each of these dishes from Phase 3 to Phase 1. Or you can order the Plain Broiled Chicken Breast or Blackened Chicken along with some vegetable side dishes to make your own combination.

RECOMMENDED DISHES

CHICKEN AND FISH DINNERS

Menu Item	Calories	Fat (g)	Sat. Fat (g)	Carbs (g)	Fiber (g)	Phase
Baked Chicken Dinner (1 piece)*	350	4	0.5	49	5	3
Baked Fish Dinner (3 pieces)*	390	5	0	49	5	3
Baked Salmon Dinner (1 piece)*	470	8	0	58	5	3

*Nutritional analysis includes rice pilaf. Eliminating the rice pilaf reduces carbohydrates, fat, and calories in this dish.

continued

CHICKEN AS A SIDE DISH

Menu Item	Calories	Fat (g)	Sat. Fat (g)	Carbs (g)	Fiber (g)	Phase
Blackened Chicken (3 pieces)	343	7	n/a	7	n/a	1
Plain Broiled Chicken Breast (1 breast)	100	1	n/a	1	0	1

VEGETABLE SIDE DISHES

Menu Item	Calories	Fat (g)	Sat. Fat (g)	Carbs (g)	Fiber (g)	Phase
Green Beans	90	3	1	15	4	1
Steamed Broccoli	25	0.5	0	5	3	1
Tuscan Vegetables	30	0	0	7	2	2

—∿— Carl's Jr. —∿—

More than 1,000 restaurants in the West
(877) 799-7827, www.carlsjr.com

It's hard to believe that this chain, which features menu items such as the massive Six Dollar Burger, began as a hot dog stand in 1941 in Los Angeles. By 1946, however, Carl Karcher, the chain's founder, was selling hamburgers at a drive-in restaurant, and burgers have been the main offering ever since. Today hamburgers are such a central part of the Carl's Jr. menu that they even offer a breakfast burger. And why does the chain call itself Carl's Jr.? Because the original two restaurants, opened in 1956, were junior versions of Carl's larger drive-in restaurants.

BEST CHOICES

South Beach dieters will find it hard but not impossible to eat at this chain. The burgers at Carl's Jr. are charbroiled and gigantic, and even the bunless version that comes wrapped in lettuce leaves is still high in fat. A better option would be the Charbroiled Chicken Salad-To-Go. Hold the grated cheese and croutons, and choose any dressing except the Thousand Island and fat-free French (12 grams of added sugar!).

The only other real choice is the Garden Salad-To-Go, a simple lettuce salad with cherry tomatoes and cucumber (hold the croutons and choose an appropriate dressing).

Some Carl's Jr. restaurants have self-serve salad bars. Be careful here—the lettuce and other vegetables are fine, but you can easily go off the South Beach Diet with additions such as pasta salad, croutons, cold cuts, and so on.

Today many Carl's Jr. restaurants also co-brand with the Green Burrito line of Mexican foods. None of the tacos, burritos, and other choices found on this portion of the menu are acceptable for South Beach dieters.

RECOMMENDED DISHES

SALADS

Menu Item	Calories	Fat (g)	Sat. Fat (g)	Carbs (g)	Fiber (g)	Phase
Charbroiled Chicken Salad-To-Go (no dressing)	330	7	4	17	5	1
Garden Salad-To-Go (no dressing)	120	3	1.5	5	2	1

—∿— Carrabba's Italian Grill —∿—

More than 168 restaurants nationwide
(813) 288-8286, www.carrabbas.com

NOTE: Nutritional information was not available for this establishment. However, we have provided some Best Choices that fit in with the South Beach Diet nutritional principles. Because we do not have specific data for these dishes, talk to your server if you have questions about the ingredients in a dish, and be especially vigilant if you are on Phase 1.

The founders of Carrabba's Italian Grill are Johnny Carrabba and Damian Mandola, two Sicilians from Texas who grew up to start their restaurant chain and host the popular *Cucina* cooking show series on PBS. Carrabba's serves high-quality Italian food in a family-friendly environment that features an open kitchen and Tuscan-style décor.

continued

BEST CHOICES

As the name suggests, Carrabba's Italian Grill offers traditional Italian favorites—including some grilled entrées that are good South Beach Diet choices. Look for Grilled Salmon, Chicken Bryan (grilled chicken breast topped with goat cheese and sun-dried tomatoes), Chicken Gratella (grilled chicken breast with olive oil and herbs), Chicken Marsala, and Sirloin Marsala. Instead of garlic mashed potatoes or pasta, ask for the vegetable of the day.

The grill also plays a role in the salads at Carrabba's. Insalata Carrabba, for instance, contains mixed field greens, mozzarella, black olives, tomatoes, and grilled chicken. Insalata Fiorucci is made with mixed field greens, artichoke hearts, roasted red bell peppers, and grilled eggplant and is topped with goat cheese. And Insalata Johnny Rocco contains mixed field greens with grilled shrimp and scallops.

—ᴥ— The Cheesecake Factory —ᴥ—

Nearly 100 locations in 28 states
(818) 871-3000, www.thecheesecakefactory.com

NOTE: Nutritional information was not available for this establishment. However, we have provided some Best Choices that fit in with the South Beach Diet nutritional principles. Because we do not have specific data for these dishes, talk to your server if you have questions about the ingredients in a dish, and be especially vigilant if you are on Phase 1.

Evelyn Overton started baking and selling her famous cheesecakes in the 1940s in California, but it wasn't until 1978 that the first The Cheesecake Factory restaurant opened in Beverly Hills. It featured an eclectic menu, large portions, and, of course, Evelyn's cheesecake. The success of the restaurant made Evelyn's cheesecake even more famous, and more restaurants and more fame followed over the years. Today this chain of casual dining restaurants offers a menu with more than 200 items, to say nothing of over 50 varieties of cheesecake.

BEST CHOICES

Even though the menu at The Cheesecake Factory is appealing, it's not that easy to find good South Beach Diet options. Among the appetizers, check out the French Country Salad, made with mixed greens, grilled asparagus, fresh beets (hold them for Phases 1 and 2), and goat cheese—just ask them to hold the candied pecans. The extensive specialties section of the menu offers a large handful of South Beach Diet–friendly entrées. Several of the chicken dishes, such as Crusted Chicken Romano, Chicken Brochettes, and Lemon-Herb Roasted Chicken, are good choices. In the fish section, look for Herb-Crusted Filet of Salmon, Miso Salmon, and Shrimp Scampi. When ordering chicken or fish entrées, substitute extra veggies for the mashed potatoes, rice, or pasta that accompany the dish. Among the main-course salads, Chicken Caesar without the croutons is a dependable choice. The Herb-Crusted Salmon Salad is another good option, and the Cobb Salad is acceptable if you hold the bacon.

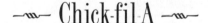

Chick-fil-A

More than 1,200 restaurants in 38 states and Washington, DC
(800) 232-2040, www.chick-fil-a.com

The unusual name of this restaurant chain dates back to its founding in 1963 by Truett Cathy. The owner of a small restaurant in Atlanta at the time, Cathy developed a way to coat boneless chicken breasts with his own breading recipe and then pressure cook them. His formula was a local success, and Cathy decided to trademark it. He came up with the name Chick-fil-A based on the idea that the boneless chicken breast was the quality equivalent of a beef fillet—why not call it a chicken fillet? Or a chick-fil for short? The capital A at the end was added to symbolize top quality. Today Chick-fil-A restaurants are found mostly in the Southeast, Texas, and Midwest, with some in the Northeast. The chain has outlets in many airports and is a major presence in mall food courts.

continued

BEST CHOICES

Chicken is the main ingredient at Chick-fil-A. It comes in a lot of forms, almost all of them breaded and therefore off-limits to South Beach dieters. The options that are left are few but flavorful. The best choice is the Chick-fil-A Chargrilled Chicken Sandwich—toss the bun and don't open the packet of Honey Roasted Barbeque Sauce. You can also try the Chick-fil-A Chargrilled Chicken Garden Salad or just a plain Side Salad (skip the croutons). The Southwest Chargrilled Salad is classified as Phase 3 because it has some corn in it. The rest of the salad, which features black beans, is fine on all phases. Most of the dressings are acceptable. Avoid the lower-fat choices such as light Italian and reduced-fat raspberry vinaigrette, and stay away from the dipping sauces.

RECOMMENDED DISHES

SOUPS, SALADS, AND SANDWICHES

Menu Item	Calories	Fat (g)	Sat. Fat (g)	Carbs (g)	Fiber (g)	Phase
Hearty Breast of Chicken Soup (1 cup)	140	3.5	1	18	1	2
Chargrilled Chicken Garden Salad (no dressing)	180	6	3	9	3	1
Chick-fil-A Southwest Chargrilled Salad (no dressing)	240	8	3.5	17	5	3
Chargrilled Chicken Sandwich (1 fillet, no bun)	100	2	0	1	0	1
Side Salad (no dressing)	60	3	1.5	4	2	1

—∞— Chili's Grill and Bar —∞—

Nearly 900 restaurants nationwide
(800) 983-4637, www.chilis.com

Chili's is one of the largest fast-casual chains, with multiple restaurants in nearly every state. The lively, family-friendly atmosphere, full bar, and varied menu make this chain one of the most popular as well.

BEST CHOICES

Some of the better-known menu items at Chili's, such as the Awesome Blossom onion (a batter-dipped fried onion served with a special sauce) are obviously a problem for South Beach dieters. Other dishes are also to be avoided, though the menu can fool you. Chili's offers what they call the Guiltless Grill, with dishes that are supposedly healthier. Read the descriptions carefully, however, and you'll realize that almost all these dishes are still way too high in refined carbs. The only dish on this part of the menu that is acceptable is the Guiltless Grill Salmon, which is served with steamed veggies and black beans.

Fortunately, there are some other dishes found elsewhere on the menu that are also fine. Try the Grilled Salmon with Garlic and Herbs or Chili's Classic Sirloin—in all cases, ask for extra veggies or a side salad instead of the rice or garlic toast they come with. The salad section of Chili's menu also has some interesting options. Lettuce Wraps (you get two, so consider sharing one) containing grilled Asian-spiced chicken (along with carrots, water chestnuts, and toasted almonds) are a good choice. Holding the crispy rice noodles and the sauces makes this a Phase 2 dish. Grilled Chicken Caesar Salad is also a fine option (eliminating the croutons makes this Phase 1).

continued

RECOMMENDED DISHES

SALADS

Menu Item	Calories	Fat (g)	Sat. Fat (g)	Carbs (g)	Fiber (g)	Phase
Grilled Chicken Caesar Salad (with croutons)	490	21	4	35	6	3
Lettuce Wraps (2)*	580	35	5	55	8	3

*Nutritional analysis includes crispy fried noodles and peanut and sesame ginger sauces. Eliminating all these reduces carbohydrates, fat, and calories in this dish.

ENTRÉES (no side dishes)

Menu Item	Calories	Fat (g)	Sat. Fat (g)	Carbs (g)	Fiber (g)	Phase
Chili's Classic Sirloin (8 oz)	530	41	14	1	0	1
Grilled Salmon with Garlic and Herbs (8 oz fillet with veggies, no rice)	412	20	3	11	4	2
Guiltless Grill Salmon (8 oz fillet with black beans and veggies)	480	14	3	31	10	2
Black Bean Burger (no bun)	200	2	0	25	20	1
Old Time Burger (no bun, no toppings)	360	25	10	0	0	3

SIDE DISHES

Menu Item	Calories	Fat (g)	Sat. Fat (g)	Carbs (g)	Fiber (g)	Phase
Black Beans (5 oz)	140	1	0	23	6	1
Steamed Veggies	90	6	1	7	3	2
Corn (without butter)	180	2	0	55	3	3

~~ Chipotle Mexican Grill ~~

More than 300 locations nationwide
(303) 595-4000, www.chipotle.com

NOTE: *Because dishes are prepared to your specifications at Chipotle Mexican Grill, we have not included nutritional information. However, we have provided some Best Choices that fit in with the South Beach Diet nutritional principles. Because we do not have specific data for these dishes, talk to your server if you have questions about the ingredients in a dish, and be especially vigilant if you are on Phase 1.*

The look and sound of a Chipotle Mexican Grill is definitely distinct. Each restaurant in this chain has its own variation on the basic décor of polished steel tables, blond wood chairs, leather stools, and red concrete floors. The music is the chain's own mix, played at a high decibel level. Many of the ingredients for the food come from small family farms.

BEST CHOICES

Chipotle offers high-quality, fast Mexican food, with an emphasis on fresh ingredients. The options for South Beach dieters, however, are limited to the Bol Salads, which are basically fajita makings served in a plastic bowl, without the tortillas and with romaine lettuce instead of rice. Go for the Grilled Chicken, Grilled Steak, or Vegetarian Bols, which include fajita veggies and guacamole; and top them with fresh tomato or tomatillo salsa. You can also order shredded Braised Pork (carnitas) or Spicy Shredded Beef (barbacoa) as side dishes, along with peppers, onions, and other fajita vegetables. Ask the server not to be too heavy handed.

—∞— Chuck E. Cheese's —∞—

More than 500 locations nationwide
(972) 258-8507, www.chuckecheese.com

The average family with children under 12 will visit a Chuck E. Cheese's restaurant five times a year. If you're that average parent and also happen to be following the South Beach Diet, chances are that now and then you'll find yourself singing along with the animated characters while wondering what you're going to be able to eat.

BEST CHOICES

The featured attraction on a typical Chuck E. Cheese's menu is pizza, pizza, and more pizza. This means your South Beach Diet options are very limited, even with the salad bar found in every restaurant. The best choices you have are a small slice of the Vegetarian or Cheese Pizza (if you're on Phase 2 or 3). If you do supplement with a trip to the salad bar, be sure to avoid the French and Thousand Island dressings, and be careful about the toppings you choose. Even your drink options are limited—the only diet soda on the menu is Diet Coke.

Trips to Chuck E. Cheese's are generally made for special occasions, like a child's birthday. If you know an expedition to this kids' paradise is coming up, try to plan your meals that day so that you can eat something at home before you get to the restaurant. That way you can skip the food or be satisfied with a small amount—and you'll have more time to play the arcade games.

RECOMMENDED DISHES

PIZZA

Menu Item	Calories	Fat (g)	Sat. Fat (g)	Carbs (g)	Fiber (g)	Phase
Vegetarian Pizza (small slice)	194	6	2	30	2	**2**
Cheese Pizza (small slice)	192	6	2	27	1	**2**

—⌇— Corner Bakery Café —⌇—

Nearly 100 locations in California, Colorado, District of Columbia,
Georgia, Illinois, Maryland, Pennsylvania, Texas, Virginia
(800) 983-4637, www.cornerbakery.com

Casual, quick, and inexpensive, Corner Bakery Cafés are a good option
for South Beach dieters in a hurry. This chain is proud of its artisanal
breads, so sandwiches are a major draw, and it also offers a good selection of interesting soups and salads for lunch and dinner. Corner Bakery
Cafés are found in some major airports, making this chain a South
Beach oasis in the wilderness of airport food courts.

BEST CHOICES

Soups at Corner Bakery Cafés vary daily. Choosing a soup to begin
your meal will help fill you up and keep you from overeating. If you're
in the mood for a salad, a good bet is the Chicken Caesar. A real bar-
gain is the Trio Salad Combination. You can get smaller portions of
any three main course salads, such as Tuna Salad, D.C. Chicken Salad,
and Tomato Fresca Salad, along with mixed greens. If you're on Phase
2 or 3, try the Corner Combo: a cup of soup or a small salad with half
a sandwich. For your sandwich half, have the Turkey Derby served on
whole-grain harvest toast.

RECOMMENDED DISHES

SOUPS AND SANDWICHES

Menu Item	Calories	Fat (g)	Sat. Fat (g)	Carbs (g)	Fiber (g)	Phase
Roasted Tomato Basil Soup (10 oz)	160	5	n/a	27	3	**2**
Spring Asparagus Soup (10 oz)	260	18	n/a	18	2	**3**
Turkey Derby (½ sandwich)*	310	8.5	n/a	31	6	**3**

*Nutritional analysis includes Swiss cheese and Thousand Island dressing. Eliminating
these reduces carbohydrates, fat, and calories in this dish.

continued

SALADS (no dressing)

Menu Item	Calories	Fat (g)	Sat. Fat (g)	Carbs (g)	Fiber (g)	Phase
Caesar Salad with Roasted Chicken (no croutons)	530	42	n/a	11	5	1
D.C. Chicken Salad (no croutons)	500	42	n/a	16	3	1
Tuna Salad	370	28	n/a	3	2	1
Tomato Fresca (with mozzarella)	200	15	n/a	10	0	3

—⚬— Cracker Barrel —⚬—
Old Country Store

More than 525 stores in 41 states
(800) 333-9566, www.crackerbarrel.com

NOTE: Nutritional information was not available for this establishment. However, we have provided some Best Choices that fit in with the South Beach Diet nutritional principles. Because we do not have specific data for these dishes, talk to your server if you have questions about the ingredients in a dish, and be especially vigilant if you are on Phase 1.

The very first Cracker Barrel Old Country Store was opened in the little town of Lebanon, Tennessee, in 1969. Founder Dan Evins wanted to start a place where travelers on the interstate road system could get gas, a good meal, and a gift in a friendly atmosphere—a place like the country stores of his childhood. The country store concept caught on, though the gas part was quickly dropped, and today the average store in the chain welcomes 1,000 or more guests a day. The homestyle cooking remains the major attraction for hungry travelers.

BEST CHOICES

The broad selection of country dishes at Cracker Barrel includes a fair number of South Beach Diet–friendly items. Eggs, country ham, and turkey sausage are all good choices from the all-day breakfast menu. You can also order Eggstro'dinaire egg substitute.

The lunch and dinner menus offer a lot of good choices. From the Fancy Fixins section, the Grilled Sirloin Steak, Grilled Chicken Tenderloin, and Lemon Pepper Grilled Trout are the best options. From the Country Dinner Plates portion of the menu, look for the Grilled Pork Chop, Grilled Chicken Tenderloin, or Spicy Catfish Fillet. Forgo the vegetable side dishes listed on the menu, and choose a small salad instead (with dressing on the side). Also skip the signature buttermilk biscuits and corn muffins. For a lighter meal, choose the Grilled Chicken Salad, skipping the wedge of Colby cheese and the accompanying croutons.

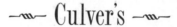

Culver's

More than 300 restaurants in 15 states
(608) 643-7980, www.culvers.com

Culver's restaurants may be best known for their famous ButterBurger, but this Midwestern chain offers a varied menu of freshly prepared food with some good South Beach Diet–compatible choices. The chain has a good reputation for cleanliness, hospitality, and a family-friendly atmosphere. Dine-in with table service or use the convenient drive-up window.

BEST CHOICES

ButterBurger Classics are burgers made from fresh beef and served on a lightly buttered, toasted bun. They come in many variations, mostly with cheese of some sort, and are fine only if you stick to the single hamburger and skip the buttered bun. Some of the sandwiches on the menu, such as the Grilled Chicken Breast or Beef Pot Roast, are also okay if you're on Phase 3. If you remove the bun or bread, these menu items become Phase 1. For all South Beach Diet phases, look for the good choice of salads, such as the Garden Fresco (hold the cheese) or the Tossed Tuna Salad. You can enjoy soup at Culver's, but be aware that the Chicken Gumbo contains rice and the Vegetable Beef with Barley Soup includes potatoes and corn. These additions make both of these soups Phase 3. The George's Chili is also fine if you're on Phase 3.

RECOMMENDED DISHES

BURGERS AND SANDWICHES

Menu Item	Calories	Fat (g)	Sat. Fat (g)	Carbs (g)	Fiber (g)	Phase
ButterBurger (single)*	346	15	6	35	1	3
Beef Pot Roast Sandwich*	307	10	3	33	1	3
Grilled Chicken Breast Sandwich*	375	8	3	47	2	3
Turkey Stacked Sandwich*	463	20	4	47	2	3
Turkey Reuben Sandwich*	401	15	5	41	2	3

*Nutritional analysis includes bun or bread. Eliminating these reduces carbohydrates, fat, and calories in this dish.

SALADS

Menu Item	Calories	Fat (g)	Sat. Fat (g)	Carbs (g)	Fiber (g)	Phase
Garden Fresco	187	9	5	23	8	1
Tossed Tuna Salad	399	25	6	11	4	1
Side Caesar (no croutons)	64	4	2	3	1	1
Side Salad	76	5	3	6	2	1

SOUPS AND STEWS

Menu Item	Calories	Fat (g)	Sat. Fat (g)	Carbs (g)	Fiber (g)	Phase
Chicken Gumbo (1 cup)	141	6	1	17	3	3
Vegetable Beef with Barley Soup (1 cup)	120	4	1	15	3	3
George's Chili (1 cup)	294	13	6	22	6	3

—ᴡ— Dairy Queen —ᴡ—

More than 5,700 locations in the US, Canada, and 22 countries
(952) 830-0200, www.dairyqueen.com

Okay, the main reason to go to a Dairy Queen is for the milkshakes, soft-serve ice cream, and other frozen treats. In fact, at some Dairy Queens (including the 600+ locations in Texas alone), that's all you can get. But don't necessarily feel you have to skip this chain. At DQs that offer the Brazier menu, you can even find a limited selection of more substantial food.

BEST CHOICES

Like many quick-serve restaurants today, DQ allows you to substitute grilled chicken for crispy chicken and a side salad for french fries. That means you're pretty much limited to the Grilled Chicken Sandwich minus the bun. Skip the honey mustard dressing (and any of the fat-free dressings, and ask for ranch on the side). If you can't face another chicken meal, your only other DQ option is the plain Homestyle Burger without the bun.

RECOMMENDED DISHES

SALADS, SANDWICHES, AND BURGERS

Menu Item	Calories	Fat (g)	Sat. Fat (g)	Carbs (g)	Fiber (g)	Phase
Grilled Chicken Salad	240	5	4	12	4	1
Grilled Chicken Sandwich (with bun)*	340	16	2	26	2	3
DQ Homestyle Burger (with bun)*	290	12	5	29	2	3
Side Salad (no dressing)	60	3	0	6	2	1

*Nutritional analysis includes bun. Eliminating the bun reduces carbohydrates, fat, and calories in this dish.

—ᴚ— Del Taco —ᴚ—

More than 400 restaurants in 14 states
(800) 852-7204, www.deltaco.com

The second-largest chain of quick-serve Mexican restaurants in the United States, Del Taco dates back to a single restaurant in Barstow, California, opened in 1964. In recent years the chain has remodeled its restaurants, giving them a modern, family-friendly design. The drive-thru window remains, but the restaurants now have expanded seating.

BEST CHOICES

A restaurant that offers Macho Combo Meals is one where South Beach dieters have to be choosy. Even the small combo meals are off-limits. Unfortunately, because this chain also specializes in hamburgers and french fries, there's not much else on the menu that's acceptable. Select the Chicken Taco del Carbon or Steak Taco del Carbon, which include grilled chicken or steak, onions, fresh cilantro, and an Anaheim chile sauce. Or try the Carnitas Taco made with pork. Removing the corn tortilla and eating only the filling makes these dishes Phase 1 rather than Phase 3. Stay away from the taco salads. Even removing the fried taco bowl still leaves you with an overly generous filling that isn't recommended for South Beach dieters.

RECOMMENDED DISHES

TACOS AND TACO SALADS

Menu Item	Calories	Fat (g)	Sat. Fat (g)	Carbs (g)	Fiber (g)	Phase
Chicken Taco del Carbon*	170	5	1	19	2	3
Carnitas Taco (pork)*	170	6	2	18	2	3
Steak Taco del Carbon*	220	11	4	19	2	3

*Nutritional analysis includes tortilla. Eliminating the tortilla reduces carbohydrates, fat, and calories in this dish.

—✖— Denny's —✖—

More than 1,600 locations nationwide
(800) 733-6697, www.dennys.com

One of the largest full-service restaurant chains, Denny's offers a menu that's reasonably South Beach Diet–friendly—and available around the clock. This chain has been a leader in offering healthier menus, and vegetarians can find something more than salads. It's also a place where it's easy to eat a good South Beach Diet breakfast.

BEST CHOICES

For breakfast, Denny's offers a wide variety of omelets made with eggs and egg substitutes. Most of these include high-fat meats such as bacon or sausage that you should be avoiding, but the Veggie-Cheese Omelet (hold the full-fat cheese if you're on Phase 1 or 2) is a good choice if you don't want just plain eggs or egg substitute. Ask them to hold the hash browns or grits, and request whole-wheat toast. Eat just one slice— but only if you're on Phase 2 or beyond. Grapefruit and Oatmeal are also available at breakfast and are acceptable if you're on Phase 2 or 3.

For lunch, try one of their filling soups before you order anything else. If you're on Phase 1 or 2, you'll have to watch out for the ones with noodles, potatoes, rice, or corn. Then look at the salad menu. The Chef Salad, Grilled Chicken Breast Salad, and Turkey Breast Salad are all acceptable. The sandwiches and melts are pretty much off-limits. The only possibility here is the Grilled Chicken Sandwich minus the bun. Alternatively, you could have a plain burger without the bun or, if you prefer, a Boca Burger without the bun. (Boca Burgers are a meatless combination of soy, spices, and cheese.) Ask for a garden salad instead of the fries, and select from the ranch, Caesar, or Italian dressings.

The dinner menu at Denny's starts at 11:00 a.m. Soup may still be available, but watch the other appetizers—there's little here that works for the South Beach Diet. As far as entrées go, stick with the Grilled Tilapia or the Grilled Chicken. Although dinners come with your choice of two sides, the selection is unfortunately very limited for South Beach dieters. Tomato slices, Green Beans, and a side Garden Salad are pretty much your only options.

continued

RECOMMENDED DISHES

BREAKFAST

Menu Item	Calories	Fat (g)	Sat. Fat (g)	Carbs (g)	Fiber (g)	Phase
Grapefruit Half	60	0	0	16	6	2
Oatmeal	100	2	0	18	3	2
Veggie-Cheese Omelet	494	39	12	11	2	3
Veggie-Cheese Omelet (Eggbeaters)	346	22	7	11	3	3
Eggbeaters (scrambled)	56	0	0	2	0	1

LUNCH

Menu Item	Calories	Fat (g)	Sat. Fat (g)	Carbs (g)	Fiber (g)	Phase
Vegetable Beef Soup (8 oz)	79	1	1	11	2	3
Chicken Noodle Soup (8 oz)	118	5	2	14	0	3
Boca Burger (with bun)*	452	11	3	64	9	3
Classic Burger (with bun)*	694	35	12	56	4	3
Caesar Salad (with croutons)*	362	26	7	20	3	3
Chef Salad (no dressing)	365	16	7	14	4	1
Garden Salad (no dressing)	113	7	5	6	2	1
Grilled Chicken Breast Salad (no dressing)	259	11	5	10	4	1
Turkey Breast Salad (no dressing)	248	8	4	12	4	1
Grilled Chicken Sandwich (with bun)*	476	14	3	56	4	3

*Nutritional analysis includes bun or croutons. Eliminating these reduces carbohydrates, fat, and calories in this dish.

DINNER

Menu Item	Calories	Fat (g)	Sat. Fat (g)	Carbs (g)	Fiber (g)	Phase
Grilled Chicken	314	8	3	8	3	1
Grilled Tilapia	300	11	3	11	3	1
Green Beans	40	1	0	8	3	1
Tomatoes	13	0	0	3	1	1

—∿— Domino's Pizza —∿—

More than 7,500 stores in more than 50 countries
(734) 930 3030, www.dominos.com

Every day more than one million people eat pizza from Domino's. This amounts to the chain selling more than 400 million pizzas a year worldwide. Looked at another way, it works out to one whole pizza plus a slice for every single person in America each year. That's a heck of a lot of pizza, especially for a chain that began as just one store in Ypsilanti, Michigan. In 1960 founder Tom Monaghan and his brother James purchased the store using $500 Tom had borrowed. In 1961 James traded his half of the business to Tom for a VW Beetle. James drove off, and Tom Monaghan went on to be a pioneer in the pizza delivery business.

BEST CHOICES

As a South Beach dieter, can you enjoy the convenience of a home-delivered pizza from Domino's? Yes, but only if you stick to the Crunchy Thin Crust pizza and customize your toppings to meet South Beach Diet recommendations. You'll have to stick to the vegetarian choices to avoid the fat-laden pepperoni and other meat toppings. That means selecting either the Green Pepper, Onion, and Mushroom Pizza or the Vegi Feast Pizza. Choose the 12-inch medium pizza, and remember that a serving is just one-eighth of a pizza, which you can have once in a while on Phase 2 or 3.

continued

RECOMMENDED DISHES

CRUNCHY THIN CRUST PIZZAS (⅛ of a 12-inch pie)

Menu Item	Calories	Fat (g)	Sat. Fat (g)	Carbs (g)	Fiber (g)	Phase
Cheese Pizza	137	7	2.5	14	1	2
Cheese Pizza with Ham	148	8	3	14	1	2
Green Pepper, Onion, and Mushroom Pizza	142	8	2.5	14	1	2
Vegi Feast Pizza	168	10	4	15	1	2

—∽— Don Pablo's —∽—

More than 100 locations in 19 states
(800) 372-2567, www.donpablos.com

One of the newer fast-casual chains, Don Pablo's has its roots in the Tex-Mex culinary tradition of Lubbock, Texas. The original restaurant, opened in 1985, was inspired by the traditional dishes of Mexican ranch cooks, which were made from scratch using fresh ingredients. Today Don Pablo's has expanded to more than 100 locations, mostly on the East Coast and in the Midwest.

BEST CHOICES

The Don Pablo's chain of Mexican restaurants is one of the few to adapt some traditional entrées for those following the South Beach Diet guidelines. In particular, Don Pablo's offers fajitas that are wrapped in lettuce, not the traditional flour tortilla. The Smoked Chicken Fajitas, Mahi Mahi Fajitas, and Black Angus Sirloin Fajitas feature grilled vegetables, such as yellow squash, zucchini, mushrooms, and asparagus— all fine on every phase of the diet. Skip the accompaniments. If you wish, you can add Grilled Shrimp to any dish. For a simpler meal or snack, order the Fresh Guacamole or the Chicken Chili Soup.

RECOMMENDED DISHES

APPETIZERS AND SALADS

Menu Item	Calories	Fat (g)	Sat. Fat (g)	Carbs (g)	Fiber (g)	Phase
Fresh Guacamole (1.25 oz)	83	8	1	4	2	1
Chicken Chili Soup (6 oz)	234	13	3	23	4	1

LETTUCE-WRAP FAJITAS (no accompaniments)

Menu Item	Calories	Fat (g)	Sat. Fat (g)	Carbs (g)	Fiber (g)	Phase
Black Angus Sirloin Fajitas	380	18.5	8	11	3	1
Mahi Mahi Fajitas	250	3.5	2	11	3	1
Smoked Chicken Fajitas	195	3.5	2	11	0	1
Grilled Shrimp (add to any dish)	127	7	1	0	0	1

—ᴡ— El Pollo Loco —ᴡ—

More than 300 restaurants in California, Arizona, Nevada, and Texas
(949) 399-2000, www.elpolloloco.com

El Pollo Loco—the crazy chicken—is a rarity among quick-service restaurants: Its main offering of grilled chicken is actually a good choice for South Beach dieters. Another unusual aspect of this chain is that it began in Mexico in 1975 with a roadside stand and expanded there first. The first US location was opened in 1980 in Los Angeles. Today most of the restaurants are located in California, with some in Arizona, Nevada, and Texas. A final notable fact about this chain: In 1995, El Pollo Loco earned a place in the *Guinness Book of World Records* for building the world's largest burrito. The feat took place on July 31 in Anaheim. The burrito was 3,112 feet long and weighed 2 tons; it took 240 volunteers 26 minutes to complete. (No word on how many people it served or how long it took to eat it.)

continued

BEST CHOICES

Chicken marinated in a special recipe of herbs, spices, and citrus juices then flame-grilled is the featured item at El Pollo Loco. This is a very South Beach Diet–friendly dish, especially if you choose breast meat. If you're on Phase 1 or 2, you'll have to turn down the corn tortillas; or you can enjoy one occasionally if you're on Phase 3. The chicken meals come with a choice of two sides. The best options are the Garden Salad, Mixed Fresh Vegetables, Pinto Beans, or Guacamole. All the salsas are acceptable. The only chicken salads you can eat at El Pollo Loco are the Caesar Pollo Salad or the Monterey Pollo Salad. The special house dressings—creamy chipotle and creamy cilantro—are fine on the side, as is the ranch dressing, but avoid the lite creamy cilantro and the Thousand Island.

RECOMMENDED DISHES

SALADS

Menu Item	Calories	Fat (g)	Sat. Fat (g)	Carbs (g)	Fiber (g)	Phase
Caesar Pollo Salad (no dressing)	221	9	2	15	4	1
Monterey Pollo Salad (no dressing)	176	6	1	12	3	1

ENTRÉES

Menu Item	Calories	Fat (g)	Sat. Fat (g)	Carbs (g)	Fiber (g)	Phase
Flame-Grilled Chicken Breast (skin removed)	153	4	1	0	0	1
Chicken Soft Taco*	237	11	5	18	1	3
Taco al Carbon (beef)*	134	3	1	18	1	3

*Nutritional analysis includes tortilla. Eliminating the tortilla reduces carbohydrates, fat, and calories in this dish.

SIDE DISHES

Menu Item	Calories	Fat (g)	Sat. Fat (g)	Carbs (g)	Fiber (g)	Phase
Garden Salad (no dressing)	77	7	1	3	1	1
Mixed Fresh Vegetables	68	4	1	6	4	1
Pinto Beans	154	4	0	24	9	1
Guacamole (2 oz)	51	3	0	5	0	1

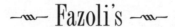

—✺— Fazoli's —✺—

More than 380 restaurants in 32 states
(859) 268-1668, www.fazolis.com

As a general rule, South Beach dieters need to avoid regular pasta (pasta that's not whole wheat or spelt). This can certainly limit your choices in an Italian restaurant, but at the Fazoli's chain, genuine whole-wheat pasta and low-fat sauces are on the menu along with some good chicken and Caesar salads.

BEST CHOICES

Salads are a good way to go if you're on Phase 1 of the South Beach Diet. An appetizer salad will fill you and make you less inclined to overdo on the pasta portions. You can also order a main course Chicken Caesar Salad without the croutons. Doing so takes this from a Phase 3 dish to a Phase 1 dish.

The best part about Fazoli's is that the chain allows diners the opportunity to build their own pasta dishes. Select a small portion of whole-wheat penne (even the small pasta portions here are huge, so take some home), add marinara sauce, and then choose a healthy topping such as roasted pepper, broccoli, or shrimp blend, tomato bruschetta mix (which does not include bread), or peppery chicken strips.

continued

RECOMMENDED DISHES

SALADS (no dressing)

Menu Item	Calories	Fat (g)	Sat. Fat (g)	Carbs (g)	Fiber (g)	Phase
Chicken Caesar Salad (with croutons)*	200	7	1.5	14	4	3
Grilled Chicken Salad	100	2	0	6	4	1
Garden Side Salad	25	0	0	4	3	1
Caesar Side Salad (with croutons)*	110	5	1	12	2	3

*Nutritional analysis includes croutons. Eliminating the croutons reduces carbohydrates, fat, and calories in this dish.

BUILD YOUR OWN PASTA

Menu Item	Calories	Fat (g)	Sat. Fat (g)	Carbs (g)	Fiber (g)	Phase
Whole-Wheat Penne, small (marinara sauce)*	480	3	0	93	11	2
Whole-Wheat Penne, small (marinara sauce, broccoli blend)*	525	5	0	98	14	2
Whole-Wheat Penne, small (marinara sauce, shrimp blend)*	560	5	0	94	11	2
Whole-Wheat Penne, small (marinara sauce, peppery chicken strips)*	550	3.5	0	94	11	2
Whole-Wheat Penne, small (marinara sauce, roasted pepper blend)*	560	6.5	0.5	101	12	2
Whole-Wheat Penne, small (marinara sauce, tomato bruschetta mix)*	525	6	0.5	95	11	2

*Small portions at Fazoli's are quite large. Reduce carbohydrates and calories by cutting back on the pasta before adding toppings.

─∾─ Friendly's ─∾─

More than 450 restaurants in 16 states
(800) 966-9970, www.friendlys.com

From the very start in Springfield, Massachusetts, back in 1935, Friendly's has been famed for two things: hamburgers and ice cream. Although the menu has expanded quite a bit since then, hamburgers and ice cream are still mainstays.

BEST CHOICES

The menu at Friendly's is heavy on breaded and fried items, melts, and burgers. There are a few South Beach Diet–friendly menu items here, however. These include a small Garden Salad, which is a good way to start your meal. There's also a Grilled Chicken Salad. Skip the fat-free dressing. As for entrées, try the meatless Gardenburger or the Grilled Chicken Deluxe (both come on a whole-wheat roll, which you can have if you're on Phase 2 or 3). If you're having breakfast at Friendly's, enjoy eggs any way you like them.

RECOMMENDED DISHES

SALADS

Menu Item	Calories	Fat (g)	Sat. Fat (g)	Carbs (g)	Fiber (g)	Phase
Garden Salad	50	2	0.5	7	1	1
Grilled Chicken Salad (with dressing)	370	10	10	20	3	3

ENTRÉES

Menu Item	Calories	Fat (g)	Sat. Fat (g)	Carbs (g)	Fiber (g)	Phase
Gardenburger (on whole-wheat roll)	560	20	4	86	10	2
Grilled Chicken Deluxe (on whole-wheat roll)	680	33	5.5	62	5	2

—⚬⚬⚬— Godfather's Pizza —⚬⚬⚬—

More than 565 restaurants in 40 states
(800) 456-8347, www.godfathers.com

According to the National Association of Pizza Operators, approximately 3 billion pizzas are sold in the United States each year. Pizza is pretty clearly one of our favorite foods. This chain is a common site for birthday parties. Godfather's also has outlets on many college campuses and at a number of airports. Bear in mind that Godfather's Pizza delivers and that not all have dining-in facilities.

BEST CHOICES

Pizza is always a bit of a problem for South Beach dieters and can't be eaten if you're on Phase 1. The crust is typically high in refined carbs, and many of the toppings, such as pepperoni and sausage, are on the bad-fats list. Even so, if you're on Phase 2 or 3, you can enjoy a slice of Godfather's Pizza occasionally if you choose the light and crispy Thin Crust Pizza and pile on the vegetables. Godfather's Pizza makes this easy with a special Vegetarian Pizza topped with green peppers, onions, mushrooms, black olives, tomatoes, and mozzarella cheese. This is about the only thing you can eat at a Godfather's Pizza. Everything else, including the sides, is off-limits.

RECOMMENDED DISHES

THIN CRUST PIZZA

Menu Item	Calories	Fat (g)	Sat. Fat (g)	Carbs (g)	Fiber (g)	Phase
Thin Crust Vegetarian (⅛ of a medium 12-inch pie)	209	9	n/a	20	1	2
Thin Crust Vegetarian (¹⁄₁₀ of a large 14-inch pie)	227	10	n/a	21	1	2
Thin Crust Cheese (⅛ of a medium 12-inch pie)	200	9	n/a	19	0	2
Thin Crust Cheese (¹⁄₁₀ of a large 14-inch pie)	215	10	n/a	19	0	2

—∿— Hard Rock Café —∿—

More than 120 locations in over 40 countries, 47 in the US
(407) 445-ROCK, www.hardrock.com

NOTE: Nutritional information was not available for this establishment. However, we have provided some Best Choices that fit in with the South Beach Diet nutritional principles. Because we do not have specific data for these dishes, talk to your server if you have questions about the ingredients in a dish, and be especially vigilant if you are on Phase 1.

A visit to a Hard Rock Café is as much an immersion in rock 'n' roll history as it is a dining experience. This chain, with more than 120 restaurants in over 40 countries (and 47 in the United States alone), has an unparalleled memorabilia collection of over 60,000 pieces. The menu is almost an afterthought. Although the chain began in London in 1971, the food has always been casual American fare.

BEST CHOICES

Your best bet at the Hard Rock Café is a salad, but you'll need to request some changes. The Caesar Salad is available with grilled chicken breast, shrimp, tuna, or salmon (hold the croutons). The Cobb Salad comes with grilled chicken and avocado, but be sure to have them hold the bacon and cheese. The Tuscan Chicken Salad features roasted asparagus and red peppers; hold the salami. Among the entrées, the Herb Grilled Chicken Breast is a reasonable choice, as long as you request fresh vegetables instead of the garlic smashed potatoes. Ditto for the Grilled Sirloin Steak—ask for extra veggies instead of the mac and cheese side.

–ᴡ– Houlihan's –ᴡ–

More than 75 locations in 19 states
(913) 901-2500, www.houlihans.com

NOTE: Nutritional information was not available for this establishment. However, we have provided some Best Choices that fit in with the South Beach Diet nutritional principles. Because we do not have specific data for these dishes, talk to your server if you have questions about the ingredients in a dish, and be especially vigilant if you are on Phase 1.

Houlihan's is a long-standing chain founded in Kansas City back in 1972. Today its restaurants are found in many neighborhoods and shopping malls, as well as in a number of airports. The offerings are a combination of classic American dishes and dishes with an ethnic flair. Because the chefs prepare the food fresh each day using local ingredients, the menu varies slightly from restaurant to restaurant.

BEST CHOICES

Some interesting choices are available for South Beach dieters at Houlihan's. Start with Asian Lettuce Wraps (sautéed sesame chicken in crisp lettuce cups), but skip the dipping sauce. Meal-sized salad choices include the standard Grilled Chicken Caesar or Salmon Caesar (without the croutons). More interesting options are the Chicken Asian Chop Chop Salad (sautéed sesame chicken on a bed of greens with Asian vegetables) and the Oriental Grilled Chicken Salad (grilled chicken breast over fresh greens with snow peas, red onions, and red bell peppers). Ask them to hold the crispy fried wonton strips on both salads. Among the entrées, try the Grilled Rosemary Chicken, Coriander-Grilled Salmon, or KC Strip Steak. Request extra veggies or a side salad instead of potatoes.

～ Jack in the Box ～

More than 2,000 restaurants in 17 states
(800) 955-5225, www.jackinthebox.com

The best-selling item at Jack in the Box restaurants is the Jumbo Jack hamburger, so called because it was one of the largest burgers in the industry when it was introduced in 1971. The next best-selling item is the Jack in the Box taco. In fact, 600 Jack in the Box tacos are eaten every minute, for a total of 315,360,000 tacos every year. Popular as these items are, they're off-limits for South Beach dieters. Fortunately, back in 1982 Jack in the Box was also the first fast-food chain to introduce salads to go.

BEST CHOICES

At nearly 600 calories (more than 300 of them from fat), the Jumbo Jack hamburger isn't an option—even when it's served bunless. You can, however, ask for the regular-size Plain Hamburger to be served without the bun. Skip the sandwiches (the Chicken Sandwich is breaded and fried) and the tacos too. If you decide to order a Plain Hamburger or one of the pita dishes, and you're on Phase 1 or 2, Jack in the Box will happily customize your order to remove the bun or pita. They will also take out the corn from the Southwest Pita filling. You'll do even better with one of the salads, such as the Asian Chicken Salad, Chicken Caesar Salad, Chicken Club Salad, or Southwest Chicken Salad.

RECOMMENDED DISHES

BURGERS AND PITAS

Menu Item	Calories	Fat (g)	Sat. Fat (g)	Carbs (g)	Fiber (g)	Phase
Plain Hamburger (with bun)*	310	14	6	30	1	**3**
Chicken Fajita Pita (with pita and cheese)*	307	10	4.5	32	3	**3**
Southwest Pita (with pita)*	260	4.5	1	35	4	**3**

*Nutritional analysis includes bun or pita. Eliminating the bun or pita reduces carbohydrates, fat, and calories in this dish.

continued

SALADS (no dressing)

Menu Item	Calories	Fat (g)	Sat. Fat (g)	Carbs (g)	Fiber (g)	Phase
Asian Chicken Salad	140	1	0	19	5	2
Chicken Caesar Salad (no croutons)	220	8	4	10	3	1
Chicken Club Salad (no condiments)	300	15	6	13	4	1
Southwest Chicken Salad	330	13	6	30	7	3
Side Salad	60	3	1.5	5	2	1

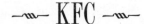

KFC

More than 11,000 restaurants in more than 80 countries
(800) 225-5532, www.kfc.com

Every year, approximately 914,000,000 pounds of chicken are served up in KFC restaurants worldwide. A lot of that chicken goes to the 26 million Americans who visit KFC restaurants over the course of a typical week. If you're a South Beach dieter, can you be one of those people? Yes, but just barely—and rarely.

BEST CHOICES

Breaded, fried foods are to be avoided when you're on the South Beach Diet, which makes your choices harder at KFC. You have to skip the Fried Chicken made with the Colonel's secret recipe of 11 herbs and spices, the Popcorn Chicken, the Chicken Strips, and anything with crunchy in the description. What does that leave? The Original Recipe Chicken Breast, which is roasted and comes without the skin and breading, or the Roasted Chicken Caesar Salad (use the ranch dressing and hold the croutons). There are also side orders of Caesar Salad, House Salad, or Green Beans.

RECOMMENDED DISHES

CHICKEN, SALADS, AND SIDES

Menu Item	Calories	Fat (g)	Sat. Fat (g)	Carbs (g)	Fiber (g)	Phase
Original Recipe Chicken Breast (roasted, no skin or breading)	140	3	1	0	0	1
Roasted Chicken Caesar Salad (no dressing, no croutons)	220	9	4.5	6	3	1
Caesar Side Salad (no dressing, no croutons)	50	3	2	2	1	1
House Side Salad (no dressing)	15	0	0	2	1	1
Green Beans	50	2	0	7	2	1

—⁓— La Salsa Fresh —⁓— Mexican Grill

More than 100 locations nationwide
(866) 527-2572, www.lasalsa.com

La Salsa restaurants are attractive, with colorful Mexican tiles, open kitchens, and fresh salsa bars. The chain began in 1979 as simple taquerias, or small neighborhood restaurants, and expanded into the fast-casual market. The menu retains the taqueria roots, however. Tacos and burritos, made with fresh ingredients and garnished with your choice of six different fresh salsas, remain the featured items.

BEST CHOICES

The emphasis on tacos, burritos, quesadillas, and other dishes makes it a little difficult to find good South Beach Diet choices on the menu. Your best bet is the tacos. By removing the tortilla, or in some cases tortillas, and eating only the shrimp, fish, or chicken filling, you can make a Phase 3 taco work for Phase 1. But even a Phase 3 dieter needs to be careful here. The tacos that come with two tortillas should be eaten only on a *very* occasional basis.

And no matter how tempting they may seem, the taco salads, which arrive in a deep-fried taco bowl, should be avoided no matter what phase of the diet you're on. Even skipping the bowl leaves you with a filling that typically contains white rice, full-fat cheese, and sour cream. In addition, South Beach dieters should resist the basket of tortilla chips that comes to the table when you sit down. Serve yourself plenty of salsa instead.

RECOMMENDED DISHES

TACOS

Menu Item	Calories	Fat (g)	Sat. Fat (g)	Carbs (g)	Fiber (g)	Phase
Baja Fish Taco (2 tortillas)*	393	25	5	30	4	3
Sonora Fish Taco (2 tortillas)*	218	10	4	17	2	3
Baja Style Shrimp Taco*	369	25	8	45	5	3
Fajita Taco with Chicken*	243	12	6	23	3	3

*Nutritional analysis includes corn tortilla(s). Eliminating the tortilla(s) reduces carbohydrates, fat, and calories in this dish.

—ᴥ— Legal Sea Foods —ᴥ—

More than 30 restaurants on the East Coast
(800) EAT FISH, www.legalseafoods.com

NOTE: Nutritional information was not available for this establishment. However, we have provided some Best Choices that fit in with the South Beach Diet nutritional principles. Because we do not have specific data for these dishes, talk to your server if you have questions about the ingredients in a dish, and be especially vigilant if you are on Phase 1.

The unusual name of this well-known chain dates back to 1950, when George Berkowitz opened a fish market next to his father's grocery store. The grocery was called Legal Cash after the "Legal Stamps" (a forerunner to S&H Green Stamps) customers were given. The name stuck to the fish market and then to the no-frills restaurant that George and his wife opened in 1968. Today, three generations of the Berkowitz family run 31 restaurants and a thriving mail-order business.

BEST CHOICES

Fish is what Legal Sea Foods is all about—and fish is what South Beach dieters should be eating, making this chain one of the easiest for finding suitable menu options. Among the appetizers, sample the classic Shrimp Cocktail or Steamed Mussels. The cold plates are slightly unusual—try the Marinated Grilled Calamari with Grilled Onions and White Beans or the Seafood Antipasto with Grilled Shrimp and Calamari (on a salad with marinated clams and mussels). Good choices among the many dinner specialty items are Cioppino (seafood and whitefish in a light tomato broth—hold the side of jasmine rice) and Spicy Grilled Tuna (ask for more spinach instead of the rice). A wide variety of wood-grilled fish and shellfish, such as tuna, sea scallops, haddock, shrimp, and seasonal specialties, is also offered. Brushed with vinaigrette or Cajun spices, the wood-grilled seafood is served with fresh vegetables and your choice of potatoes or rice—ask for extra veggies instead. For those who don't enjoy fish, sirloin steak and chicken breast are also available from the grill.

–~– Little Caesars Pizza –~–

More than 3,000 stores worldwide
(800) 722-3727, www.littlecaesars.com

You know the slogan: Pizza! Pizza! It's heavily advertised, and it's Little Caesars' memorable way of promoting the chain's famous two-for-one pizza deal. Take-out pizza is a quick, easy family meal; and if you're like most harried parents, you're going to end up eating it for dinner now and then. With care, it's possible to enjoy a slice or two.

BEST CHOICES

To minimize the amount of refined carbs you get from a Little Caesars pizza, choose the Thin Crust version. And to minimize the bad fats that come with pepperoni and sausage, stick to the veggie toppings: green peppers, onions, black olives, mushrooms, tomatoes, and a sprinkling of banana pepper rings for some extra zip. On request, Little Caesars will also make your pizza genuinely vegan—and lower in fat—by leaving off the mozzarella cheese.

Even when you've done all you can to make your pizza healthier by South Beach Diet standards, you should still limit yourself to an occasional slice (and skip it altogether on Phase 1). To round out your meal, try a Tossed, Greek, or Caesar Salad (without the croutons). Avoid the Antipasto Salad—it includes too many high-fat ingredients. All the dressings at Little Caesars are acceptable.

RECOMMENDED DISHES

THIN CRUST PIZZA

Menu Item	Calories	Fat (g)	Sat. Fat (g)	Carbs (g)	Fiber (g)	Phase
Thin Crust Veggie (⅛ of 12-inch pizza)	161	9	3	15	0	2
Thin Crust Veggie (¹⁄₁₀ of 14-inch pizza)	181	10	3.5	16	0	2

SALADS (no dressing)

Menu Item	Calories	Fat (g)	Sat. Fat (g)	Carbs (g)	Fiber (g)	Phase
Caesar Salad (no croutons)	90	3	1	12	3	1
Greek Salad	120	7	4.5	11	3	1
Tossed Salad	100	3	1	15	3	1

—∞— Lone Star —∞—
Steakhouse & Saloon

More than 200 locations in 35 states
(316) 264-8899, www.lonestarsteakhouse.com

Eating at a Lone Star Steakhouse is fun. This mid-priced chain of casual dining restaurants features a Texas roadhouse ambience, with planked wooden floors, flags, Texas memorabilia, and country-and-western music. The menu offers steak and other items served in generous, Texas-sized portions.

BEST CHOICES

For an appetizer, try the filling black bean soup (it will keep you from eating too much later). As a main course, have the mesquite-grilled steaks or chicken. Among these, the Five-Star Filet is one option; it can easily be turned into a Phase 1 dish if you ask your server to hold the bacon wrap. The large San Antonio Sirloin is also a good choice if you share or take some home. Kabobs made with grilled chicken or beef are other South Beach Diet–friendly dishes. Among the side dishes, stick with the lettuce wedge (without the dressing), Sautéed Mushrooms, or Steamed Vegetables.

continued

RECOMMENDED DISHES

APPETIZERS AND SIDE DISHES

Menu Item	Calories	Fat (g)	Sat. Fat (g)	Carbs (g)	Fiber (g)	Phase
Black Bean Soup (6 oz)	189	4	1	31	7	1
Sautéed Mushrooms	115	9	2	6	2	1
Steamed Vegetables	71	1	0	14	22	2

ENTRÉES

Menu Item	Calories	Fat (g)	Sat. Fat (g)	Carbs (g)	Fiber (g)	Phase
Five-Star Filet (9 oz)*	738	28	10	0	0	3
San Antonio Sirloin (12 oz)	768	24	10	0	0	1
Grilled Chicken (6 oz)	186	2	0.5	0	0	1
Grilled Chicken Kabob	n/a	n/a	n/a	n/a	n/a	1
Shrimp Dinner (4 oz, no rice)	103	2	0.5	1	0	1
Grilled Beef Kabob	n/a	n/a	n/a	n/a	n/a	1
Lone Star Chili with Cheese (6 oz)	228	15	6	8	1.5	3

*Nutritional analysis for this dish is with bacon wrap. Eliminating the bacon reduces fat and calories in this dish.

~~ Luby's Cafeteria ~~

More than 1,320 locations in Texas
(800) 886-4600, www.lubys.com

Generations of Texans have grown up eating at Luby's Cafeteria. This chain, founded in 1947, has become a Texas institution. If you're a South Beach dieter in Texas, that means you're in luck, because Luby's offers an unusually good selection of dishes that fit well within the guidelines.

BEST CHOICES

The Luby's menu varies some from day to day, and there are usually seasonal specials, but the basic menu always offers a good variety of South Beach Diet–friendly dishes. Look for the selection of grilled and baked fish dishes, such as the Blackened Tilapia or Lemon Basil Salmon. Other good choices include Roasted Chicken, Roasted Turkey, Grilled Chicken Breast, or a Grilled Chicken Caesar Salad without the croutons. Among the side dishes, you have your choice of a large number of vegetables, including Green Beans, Broccoli, Carrots, Cabbage, and Spinach. There's also a small Spinach Salad and Mixed Field Greens Salad on the menu (skip the honey mustard and French dressings). If you're on Phase 2 or 3, you can order Grapefruit as a side dish.

RECOMMENDED DISHES

ENTRÉES

Menu Item	Calories	Fat (g)	Sat. Fat (g)	Carbs (g)	Fiber (g)	Phase
Blackened Chicken Breast	350	15	n/a	5	2	1
Grilled Chicken Breast	400	20	n/a	1	0	1
Half Roasted Chicken (no skin)	460	23	n/a	0	0	1
Grilled Chicken Caesar Salad (no dressing)	370	13	n/a	16	6	3
Roasted Turkey (no skin)	280	3	n/a	0	0	1

continued

ENTRÉES *(continued)*

Menu Item	Calories	Fat (g)	Sat. Fat (g)	Carbs (g)	Fiber (g)	Phase
Blackened Tilapia	270	11	n/a	5	2	1
Parmesan-Crusted Tilapia	300	14	n/a	6	0	1
Lemon Basil Salmon	355	20	n/a	1	0	1

SIDE DISHES

Menu Item	Calories	Fat (g)	Sat. Fat (g)	Carbs (g)	Fiber (g)	Phase
Broccoli	80	4	n/a	9	5	1
Cabbage	70	5	n/a	6	3	1
Carrots	94	4	n/a	15	3	2
Cauliflower, Peas, and Carrots	67	4	n/a	7	3	2
Green Beans	92	5	n/a	10	5	1
Pinto Beans	190	5	n/a	28	11	1
Roasted Mixed Vegetables	135	8	n/a	16	4	1
Spinach	65	4	n/a	5	3	1
Spinach Salad (no dressing)	47	2	n/a	5	3	1
Mixed Field Greens Salad (no dressing)	34	0	n/a	7	3	1
Grapefruit	46	0	n/a	12	2	2

—∽— Marie Callender's —∽—

More than 160 locations in the Western states
(800) 776-7437, www.mcpies.com

NOTE: Nutritional information was not available for this establishment. However, we have provided some Best Choices that fit in with the South Beach Diet nutritional principles. Because we do not have specific data for these dishes, talk to your server if you have questions about the ingredients in a dish, and be especially vigilant if you are on Phase 1.

Marie Callender is probably best known for frozen foods, particularly pies—both the sweet kind and others, such as chicken pot pie. The company also operates a chain of family-friendly restaurants featuring standard American fare and, of course, freshly baked pies.

BEST CHOICES

The signature entrées at Marie Callender's, such as the Heartland Turkey Pot Pie, are off-limits if you're on the South Beach Diet. Better choices are the Fresh Catch of the Day (as long as it's not breaded and fried), the Grilled Lemon Chicken, and the Pepper-Crusted Sirloin Steak. Ask for extra veggies or a salad instead of the rice pilaf or mashed potatoes. Or head for the soup and salad bar. The homemade soups vary from day to day. Select one like Hearty Vegetable Soup, which is light on refined carbs such as noodles. The salad bar offers all the usual greens and garnishes, including fresh fruit. Choose carefully, avoiding the pasta salads, bacon, deli meats, and reduced-fat dressings, which are likely to have added sugar. Marie Callender's also offers an interesting variation on the standard Caesar Salad—you can have it topped with freshly carved roasted turkey breast but always skip the croutons. The Cabo San Lucas Chicken Salad—basically a Southwestern-style Caesar salad with grilled chicken—is a good choice as long as you skip the tortilla chips.

—ᴍ— McDonald's —ᴍ—

More than 30,000 restaurants in 119 countries
(800) 244-6227, www.mcdonalds.com

Think fast food and you can't help but think McDonald's—more than 50 million people worldwide eat at one of the chain's restaurants every day. As a South Beach dieter, can you eat there too? Yes, if you stay away from the iconic Big Mac (introduced in 1968), the french fries, Chicken McNuggets, and all the other heavily advertised choices, and instead choose one of the handful of more acceptable alternatives.

BEST CHOICES

You can always ask for a hamburger without the bun at McDonald's, and you can now request a side salad instead of fries in the combination meals. That said, we've assigned the Plain Hamburger without the bun to Phase 3 because of our concern about saturated fat. For a more interesting set of possibilities, however, look at the salad menu. McDonald's now offers several different meal-sized salads, such as the California Cobb with Grilled Chicken. With just a little work, you can tailor these salads to the SBD guidelines. First, for chicken salads, be sure to get the grilled chicken—the crispy chicken is breaded and should be avoided. Then select a dressing with no added sugar: One of the Newman's Own dressings (such as light balsamic or ranch) would be good, or you can choose light mayonnaise.

McDonald's has recently added some premium sandwiches made with chicken. As with the salads, these are fine if you're careful to order grilled, not crispy, chicken and then toss the buns and in some cases the bacon. The new Fruit and Walnut Salad at McDonald's sounds like it ought to be a great option for South Beach dieters, but the walnuts are candied, so you'll have to skip this one or eat it without the nuts.

RECOMMENDED DISHES

SALADS (no dressing)

Menu Item	Calories	Fat (g)	Sat. Fat (g)	Carbs (g)	Fiber (g)	Phase
Caesar Salad (no croutons)	90	4	2.5	9	3	1
Caesar Salad (with grilled chicken, no croutons)	220	6	3	12	3	1
California Cobb (with grilled chicken)	280	11	5	12	4	1
Fruit and Walnut Salad (no walnuts)	170	1	0.5	38	4	2
Side Salad	20	0	0	4	1	1

BURGERS AND SANDWICHES

Menu Item	Calories	Fat (g)	Sat. Fat (g)	Carbs (g)	Fiber (g)	Phase
Plain Hamburger (no bun)	100	7	3	1	0	3
Premium Grilled Chicken Classic (no bun)	180	7	1.5	2	0	1
Premium Grilled Chicken Club (no bun, no bacon)	260	13	5	5	0	1

—ᴂᴂ— Old Chicago —ᴂᴂ—

More than 85 restaurants in 20 states
(303) 664-4000, www.rockbottomrestaurantsinc.com

Old Chicago is a relatively new and expanding chain of casual restaurants. The specialty here is beer—110 varieties of it. If you sample every one (not all in one night!), you get your name inscribed in the Old Chicago Hall of Foam. Beer is not on your South Beach Diet foods-to-enjoy list, but Old Chicago does make an effort to provide some dishes that are reasonable options for people interested in healthy eating.

BEST CHOICES

Since you're not going to drink the beer or eat the deep-dish pizza at Old Chicago, what's left? Chicken. Among the entrée salads, consider the Cajun-Style Blackened Chicken Salad. Two other chicken entrées are also interesting possibilities. Chicken Rustica is a marinated grilled chicken breast served with fresh salsa and steamed fresh vegetables. The Grilled Chicken Wrap contains chicken, lettuce, tomato, red onions, and Parmesan cheese drizzled with Italian dressing and served in a whole-wheat tortilla.

RECOMMENDED DISHES

SALADS AND WRAPS

Menu Item	Calories	Fat (g)	Sat. Fat (g)	Carbs (g)	Fiber (g)	Phase
Blackened Chicken Salad*	409	12	2	19	4	3
Chicken Rustica	513	21	3	16	6	2
Grilled Chicken Wrap (with whole-wheat tortilla)	516	20	4	58	34	2
Side Caesar (with dressing and croutons)**	318	27	7	7	2	3
House Salad (no dressing)	57	2	0	7	2	1

*Nutritional analysis includes Craisins and ranch dressing. Eliminating these reduces carbohydrates, fat, and calories in this dish.

**Nutritional analysis includes croutons and dressing. Eliminating these reduces carbohydrates, fat, and calories in this dish.

—∾— Olive Garden —∾—
Italian Restaurant

More than 550 restaurants nationwide
(800) 331-2729, www.olivegarden.com

NOTE: Nutritional information was not available for this establishment. However, we have provided some Best Choices that fit in with the South Beach Diet nutritional principles. Because we do not have specific data for these dishes, talk to your server if you have questions about the ingredients in a dish, and be especially vigilant if you are on Phase 1.

Olive Garden bills itself as a genuine Italian dining experience. The chain develops its recipes and sends its managers for training at the Culinary Institute of Tuscany in Italy. The idea is to bring authentic cuisine to the restaurants and combine it with Italian-style hospitality. The slogan at Olive Garden is, "When you're here, you're family."

BEST CHOICES

The menu at Olive Garden has some dishes marked with a little olive branch symbol indicating the Garden Fare selections. These dishes are lower-fat options, but most are still not the best for South Beach dieters. Some pasta dishes are marked as low-fat, for example, but they're still way too high in refined carbs. In fact, all the pasta dishes at Olive Garden should be avoided by South Beach dieters—which means that except for the dishes mentioned here, almost all of the menu is off-limits. Some of the daily specials may be fine—ask your server about them.

Among the appetizers, the Sicilian Shrimp Scampi or the Mussels di Napoli (steamed mussels with wine, garlic butter, and onions) are both okay. For salads, the Garden-Fresh Side Salad comes with unlimited refills. The classic Grilled Chicken Caesar Salad is a good choice, as long as you hold the croutons. One of the authentic things about the Olive Garden menu is the grill—an often-forgotten aspect of Italian cooking. The best choices here are Pork Filettino (rosemary pork tenderloin) or Salmon Piccata (salmon fillet in white wine lemon sauce). Ask for extra grilled veggies or a salad instead of the Tuscan potatoes.

—∿— On the Border —∿—
Mexican Grill & Cantina

More than 130 restaurants in 31 states
(800) 983-4637, www.ontheborder.com

On the Border Mexican Grill & Cantina is a popular chain serving Mexican fare in a family-friendly, casual atmosphere. The menu is fairly extensive and has a number of grilled and seafood items—which means that South Beach dieters have a good chance of finding some allowable dishes with authentic Mexican flavor.

BEST CHOICES

For an appetizer, try the Guacamole Live!, which is made fresh to order at your table (this is a large portion for four people and is ideal for sharing). Or, for fun, there's the Shaken Margarita Shrimp Cocktail (chilled shrimp, chopped avocado, fresh jalapeños, and zesty tomato salsa are all shaken together at your table and served straight up—skip the tortilla crisps). Alternatively, have a starter salad with ranch dressing or fresh salsa.

As far as entrées go, the fajita grill offers a variety of options, including mesquite-grilled steak, chicken, shrimp, and grilled vegetables. Just skip the tortillas that come with these dishes, ask for extra black beans or grilled vegetables instead of rice, and choose guacamole instead of cheese. If you do this, the fajitas move from Phase 3 to Phase 1. The rest of the menu is largely the usual burritos, chimichangas, enchiladas, tacos, and other Mexican favorites—all dishes you'll want to skip. Even the Salmon Mexican and Mexican Shrimp Scampi, which may seem okay at first glance, are very high in fat and saturated fat, so stay away from these dishes too.

RECOMMENDED DISHES

APPETIZERS AND SALADS

Menu Item	Calories	Fat (g)	Sat. Fat (g)	Carbs (g)	Fiber (g)	Phase
Guacamole Live! (serves 4)	142	12	2.5	8	8	1
Shaken Margarita Shrimp Cocktail (no tortilla crisps)	280	11	2	24	8	1
House Salad (no dressing)	170	10	4	15	4	1

FAJITAS

Menu Item	Calories	Fat (g)	Sat. Fat (g)	Carbs (g)	Fiber (g)	Phase
Grilled Vegetable Fajitas*	390	28	3	30	7	3
Chicken Fajitas*	440	18	3	20	4	3
Steak Fajitas*	620	41	12	18	3	3

*Nutritional analysis includes tortilla. Eliminating the tortilla reduces carbohydrates, fat, and calories in this dish.

SIDE DISHES

Menu Item	Calories	Fat (g)	Sat. Fat (g)	Carbs (g)	Fiber (g)	Phase
Grilled Vegetables	50	1	0	8	3	1
Black Beans (1 cup)	180	7	2	19	8	1
Large Shrimp (4 sautéed)	170	10	4	1	0	1
Chili con Queso (1 cup)	250	18	12	8	1	3

–∞– Outback Steakhouse –∞–

More than 900 restaurants nationwide
(813) 282-1225, www.outbacksteakhouse.com

NOTE: Nutritional information was not available for this establishment. However, we have provided some Best Choices that fit in with the South Beach Diet nutritional principles. Because we do not have specific data for these dishes, talk to your server if you have questions about the ingredients in a dish, and be especially vigilant if you are on Phase 1.

The Outback Steakhouse chain has grown with amazing speed since the first restaurant was opened in 1988 in Tampa. The Australian-themed restaurants offer generous portions, moderate prices, and a casual atmosphere. Steaks and seafood are the specialties here, making this chain a good option for South Beach dieters.

BEST CHOICES

The Aussie slang on the Outback menu takes a little getting used to. The massive Bloomin' Onion is a featured Aussie-Tizer, for instance. Basically a deep-fried onion, it's not the sort of appetizer a South Beach dieter wants. The only first course you should consider is Grilled Shrimp. Among the salads, check out the Brisbane Caesar Salad, with your choice of grilled shrimp or chicken on top (skip the croutons). If you'd like a steak (and steak is the reason most people go to Outback), try Victoria's 'Center Cut' Filet, a 7-ounce tenderloin. Other lower-fat cuts include the Outback Special (9-ounce sirloin) and Ayers Rock Strip (14-ounce New York strip). If you order the big steak, share it or take some home. Ask for extra vegetables instead of the potato or Aussie chips. To find the fish selections at Outback, look under the menu heading "Botany Bay Catches." The options come down to Grilled North Atlantic Salmon and Grilled Fish of the Day—both are served with steamed vegetables.

—∽— Panda Express —∽—

More than 700 restaurants nationwide
(800) 877-8988, www.pandaexpress.com

Andrew Cherng, the founder of Panda Express, came to America from the picturesque Yangzhou region of China, bringing recipes from his father, a renowned chef, with him. Those recipes formed the basis for a chain that now has over 700 restaurants, including many in food courts, sports venues, airports, and other locations attractive to hungry, busy people.

BEST CHOICES

The best choices at Panda Express include the stir-fried dishes, such as Beef with Broccoli, Chicken with Mushrooms, and Mixed Vegetables, which are prepared in soybean oil. South Beach dieters need to avoid the white rice that comes along with stir-fried dishes from Panda Express. Also stay away from sweet-and-sour sauces, barbecue sauces, deep-fried choices such as egg rolls, and any rice or noodle-based dishes on the menu. We have labeled the dishes below as Phase 2 to take into account any possible thickening agents used during cooking. Ask your server how a particular dish is prepared.

RECOMMENDED DISHES

ENTRÉES

Menu Item	Calories	Fat (g)	Sat. Fat (g)	Carbs (g)	Fiber (g)	Phase
Beef with Broccoli	150	8	2	9	1	2
Beef with String Beans	170	9	2	11	2	2
Chicken with Mushrooms	130	7	1.5	7	2	2
Black Pepper Chicken	180	10	2	10	2	2
Mandarin Chicken	250	9	2.5	8	2	2
Mixed Vegetables	70	3	0.5	8	1	2

—ᴡᴡ— Panera Bread —ᴡᴡ—

More than 800 bakery-cafés in 35 states
(314) 633-7100, www.panerabread.com

The quick service, pleasant décor, and sandwich variety make this rapidly growing chain a favorite choice for lunch. In addition, Panera Bread bakery-cafés offer a good variety of interesting salads and soups. The You Pick Two deal lets you select any two from a choice of a bowl of soup, any half sandwich, or any half salad—an excellent approach for South Beach dieters. And if you're in a hurry, you can call or fax ahead and your order will be waiting for you.

BEST CHOICES

The soup menu at Panera Bread varies from day to day. If the Low-Fat Vegetarian Black Bean or Low-Fat Vegetarian Garden Vegetable Soup is available when you're there, you're in luck—these are both good choices. Most of the salads at Panera Bread are acceptable. Go for the basic Caesar or one with grilled chicken. If you eliminate the croutons on the Grilled Chicken Caesar, it becomes a Phase 1 dish.

Needless to say, at Panera Bread they take their store-baked artisan and specialty breads very seriously. The sandwiches on the menu are paired with particular breads, but South Beach dieters should ask only for the multigrain bread, made with nine whole grains. If you do so, a sandwich assigned to Phase 3 becomes a Phase 2. The sandwich fillings are varied and interesting. Good choices include the Asiago Roast Beef, Sierra Turkey, and Garden Veggie. Panera Bread also offers the traditional sandwich standbys: Smoked Turkey Breast, Chicken Salad, and Tuna Salad. All the sandwiches can end up being a little higher in calories, fat, and carbohydrates than you might want—take advantage of the You Pick Two option to have just a half, or share your sandwich with someone else.

RECOMMENDED DISHES

SOUPS AND SALADS (with dressing)

Menu Item	Calories	Fat (g)	Sat. Fat (g)	Carbs (g)	Fiber (g)	Phase
Low-Fat Vegetarian Black Bean Soup	160	1	0	31	11	1
Low-Fat Vegetarian Garden Vegetable Soup	90	1	0	17	2	3
Caesar Salad* (with croutons)	390	26	9	22	3	1
Classic Café Salad	390	37	5	14	4	1
Grilled Chicken Caesar Salad* (with croutons)	500	33	9	19	3	3

*Nutritional analysis includes croutons. Eliminating croutons reduces carbohydrates, fat, and calories in this dish.

SANDWICHES

Menu Item	Calories	Fat (g)	Sat. Fat (g)	Carbs (g)	Fiber (g)	Phase
Asiago Roast Beef (focaccia)*	730	35	15	54	2	3
Sierra Turkey (Asiago cheese focaccia)*	950	55	14	71	4	3
Garden Veggie (ciabatta)*	570	23	8	74	5	3
Smoked Turkey Breast (sourdough bread)*	440	15	2.5	44	3	3
Chicken Salad (multigrain bread)	640	29	5	56	4	2
Tuna Salad (multigrain bread)	830	41	6	78	5	2

*Nutritional analysis is with the bread indicated. Ask for multigrain bread instead for a Phase 2 sandwich.

~~~ Papa John's Pizza ~~~

Nearly 3,000 restaurants in 49 states
(502) 261-4275, www.papajohns.com

When a restaurant chain is named Papa John's Pizza, there has to be a real John somewhere. In the case of this company, it's founder John Schnatter. In 1984, Schnatter knocked out a broom closet in his father's tavern, sold his car to buy $1,600 worth of used restaurant equipment, and began selling his pizzas to the tavern's customers. He soon expanded into an adjoining space and opened his first Papa John's restaurant in Jeffersonville, Indiana, in 1985. Today the chain has nearly 3,000 restaurants in 49 states and 20 international markets.

BEST CHOICES

Papa John's sticks to traditional pizza, which means either a standard crust or a thin crust—no deep-dish pizza here. The restaurants break with tradition a bit to provide a more interesting choice of toppings, which are fine on the South Beach Diet. Start with a thin crust base, then select one of the lower-fat toppings: Garden Fresh Vegetable (green peppers, onions, baby portobello mushrooms, black olives, tomatoes), Spinach Alfredo, Grilled Chicken Alfredo, or Spinach Alfredo Chicken Tomato. Remember, a slice of pizza is an occasional treat, even on Phase 3. Papa John's offers online ordering and call-ahead ordering so your pizza will be ready for pickup when you arrive.

RECOMMENDED DISHES

THIN CRUST PIZZA

Menu Item	Calories	Fat (g)	Sat. Fat (g)	Carbs (g)	Fiber (g)	Phase
Garden Fresh Vegetable Pizza (⅛ of a large, 14-inch pizza)	230	12	3	25	2	**2**
Spinach Alfredo Pizza (⅛ of a large, 14-inch pizza)	240	14	4.5	21	1	**2**

Menu Item	Calories	Fat (g)	Sat. Fat (g)	Carbs (g)	Fiber (g)	Phase
Grilled Chicken Alfredo Pizza (⅛ of a large, 14-inch pizza)	250	13	4	21	1	2
Spinach Alfredo Chicken Tomato Pizza (⅛ of a large, 14-inch pizza)	250	14	4.5	22	1	2

—∿— Pei Wei Asian Diner —∿—

More than 75 locations in 13 states
(480) 888-3000, www.peiwei.com

Pan-Asian cuisine, served up quickly and eaten in the dining room or taken away, is the basic concept at Pei Wei (pronounced *Pay Way*) Asian Diner. Eat in to enjoy the sights, sounds, and smells from the open kitchen as the chefs prepare the food of Thailand, Vietnam, Japan, Korea, and China in blazing woks. This is a family-friendly restaurant with large portions that are meant to be shared—the average dish serves at least two. As with all Asian cuisine, the menu is heavy on rice and noodles, but also has a number of South Beach Diet–friendly dishes, including soups, salads, and main courses.

BEST CHOICES

Under the First Tastes section of the menu, look for the Minced Chicken in Cool Lettuce Wraps—a refreshing mix of minced chicken with shiitake mushrooms, water chestnuts, scallions, and spicy soy sauce served in a crispy lettuce wrap. Ask for the soy sauce on the side, and use only a dab of it. One salad, the Asian Chopped Chicken Salad, is also a good choice. Just hold the crispy wontons to make it suitable for Phase 1. You'll need to skip over the noodles and rice bowls and go straight to the Signature Dishes, an interesting assortment of items drawn from across Asia. The Signature Dishes are made with your choice of chicken, pork, shrimp, scallops, beef, or vegetables with tofu. Choose the ingredient you want, then select the dish you want it in. The best choices here are anything from the Mongolian or Lemon Pepper section of the menu. You can also choose the Vegetables and Tofu from the Pei Wei and Mandarin area, but skip all the other offerings. Avoid the rice, unless you're on Phase 2 or 3, when a small amount of the brown rice is acceptable. Pei Wei adds no MSG to its dishes.

RECOMMENDED DISHES

APPETIZERS, SOUPS, AND SALADS

Menu Item	Calories	Fat (g)	Sat. Fat (g)	Carbs (g)	Fiber (g)	Phase
Minced Chicken in Cool Lettuce Wraps	125	2	n/a	15	1.5	1
Edamame (soybeans)	75	4	n/a	6	2.5	1
Hot & Sour Soup (1 cup)	150	9	n/a	11	2	1
Asian Chopped Chicken Salad*	140	8	n/a	6.5	1	3

*Nutritional analysis includes crispy wontons. Eliminating the wontons reduces carbohydrates, fat, and calories in this dish.

SIGNATURE DISHES

Menu Item	Calories	Fat (g)	Sat. Fat (g)	Carbs (g)	Fiber (g)	Phase
Mongolian Chicken*	140	4.5	n/a	7	1	1
Mongolian Beef*	210	11	n/a	7	1	1
Mongolian Vegetables and Tofu*	90	3	n/a	10	2	2
Mongolian Shrimp*	105	3	n/a	6	1	1
Mongolian Scallops*	100	3	n/a	7	0	1
Pei Wei Spicy Vegetables and Tofu*	125	8	n/a	10	2	2
Mandarin Kung Pao Vegetables and Tofu*	150	8	n/a	12	2	2
Lemon Pepper Chicken*	220	10	n/a	17	2	1

Menu Item	Calories	Fat (g)	Sat. Fat (g)	Carbs (g)	Fiber (g)	Phase
Lemon Pepper Beef*	225	15	n/a	16	1	1
Lemon Pepper Vegetables and Tofu*	115	5	n/a	15	2	2
Lemon Pepper Shrimp*	190	9	n/a	17	1	1
Lemon Pepper Scallops*	180	8	n/a	17	1	1

*Pei Wei's Signature Dishes typically contain 2 servings. Nutritional analyses, above and on the opposite page, are for 1 serving, without rice.

—⚬— P.F. Chang's China Bistro —⚬—

More than 100 bistros in 32 states
(480) 888-3000, www.pfchangs.com

The cuisines of Southeast Asia are becoming increasingly popular among American diners. P.F. Chang's China Bistro, a chain of upscale casual restaurants, offers not only traditional Chinese dishes but also some menu items influenced by other Asian food traditions. All the menu items are prepared in open kitchens, allowing diners to see the wok action as the chefs cook.

BEST CHOICES

Chinese food can be a bit of a problem for South Beach dieters—many of the dishes contain rice or noodles, and the sauces are often made with cornstarch. If you're on Phase 1 of the South Beach Diet, rice is off your radar. Once you enter Phase 2, however, you can add limited amounts of brown rice to your diet. Fortunately, at P.F. Chang's brown rice is available, and many of the dishes come without rice or noodles.

The menu at P.F. Chang's is extensive; you'll have to read it carefully to find the most South Beach Diet–friendly dishes. Always skip the dumplings and lettuce wraps (which include rice sticks and a sugary sauce), and go for the Seared Ahi Tuna or the Wild Alaskan Sockeye Salmon Salad instead.

continued

The entrées at P.F. Chang's sound wonderfully appropriate for the South Beach Diet, but you'll have to ask that they be prepared with chicken broth and not with cornstarch or potato starch. This is true for the many vegetable entrées as well. Making this request would take these dishes from Phase 3 to Phase 1, and P.F. Chang's is happy to do it.

RECOMMENDED DISHES

APPETIZERS AND SALADS

Menu Item	Calories	Fat (g)	Sat. Fat (g)	Carbs (g)	Fiber (g)	Phase
Seared Ahi Tuna	220	5	1	18	n/a	1
Wild Alaskan Sockeye Salmon Salad	470	30	4	18	n/a	1

CHICKEN AND SEAFOOD ENTRÉES

Menu Item	Calories	Fat (g)	Sat. Fat (g)	Carbs (g)	Fiber (g)	Phase
Ginger Chicken and Broccoli*	620	21	2.5	43	n/a	3
Lemon Pepper Shrimp*	520	25	2.5	31	n/a	3
Cantonese Shrimp*	380	15	2	17	n/a	3
Cantonese Scallops*	370	13	1.5	20	n/a	3
Wild Alaskan Sockeye Salmon Lemon Pepper*	670	36	5	32	n/a	3

VEGETABLE ENTRÉES

Menu Item	Calories	Fat (g)	Sat. Fat (g)	Carbs (g)	Fiber (g)	Phase
Buddha's Feast (steamed)*	200	0	0	44	n/a	3
Garlic Snap Peas*	220	7	0.5	20	n/a	3
Shanghai Cucumbers*	120	6	1	8	n/a	3
Sichuan-Style Asparagus*	190	4	0.5	36	n/a	3
Spinach Stir-Fried with Garlic*	110	4	1	15	n/a	3

*Nutritional analysis is with cornstarch, potato starch, and/or oyster sauce. Ask to have these dishes prepared in chicken broth instead.

—⚬— Piccadilly —⚬—

More than 130 cafeterias in 15 states
(225) 293-9440, www.piccadilly.com

Piccadilly is one of the largest cafeteria chains in the nation, with franchises in 15 states, but primarily in the Southeast and Mid-Atlantic region. Baton Rouge, where the first Piccadilly was founded in 1944 by T.H. (Tandy) Hamilton, remains the corporate headquarters. Cafeterias in general turn out to be good dining options for South Beach dieters—the variety of food makes it easy to find something interesting and healthful to eat. Piccadilly is no exception—it strives to be a family-friendly place with a varied menu.

BEST CHOICES

The menu at Piccadilly is fairly extensive, plus there's usually a special or two on any given day. The chain's Dilly Meals come with an entrée and your choice of two sides. They're served all day and are an excellent value. Your best South Beach Diet choice is one of the fish dishes, such as Cajun Baked Bass or Cajun Baked Tilapia. Other good entrée options would be the Rotisserie Chicken Breast Quarter or the Mesquite-Smoked Chicken Breast (always remove the skin). The carved Turkey Breast is another good choice.

The salad selection is broad, with some interesting options such as Asparagus and Tomato Salad. Whatever salad you choose, have it with Italian or ranch dressing on the side. For side dishes, you can pick from an unusually wide variety of vegetables. Many of them are buttered, and some, like the collard greens, are sautéed with bacon. Skip the ones with bacon, and request those with butter to be steamed instead. This will make them suitable for Phase 1.

continued

RECOMMENDED DISHES

SEAFOOD ENTRÉES

Menu Item	Calories	Fat (g)	Sat. Fat (g)	Carbs (g)	Fiber (g)	Phase
Baked Grouper Filet (8 oz)	330	9	2	8	1	1
Baked Tilapia (8 oz)	210	11	2	10	1	1
Baked Trout Filet (8 oz)	464	19	4	10	1	1
Cajun Baked Bass (8 oz)	263	15	4	4	1	1
Cajun Baked Tilapia (8 oz)	267	19	4	7	2	1

POULTRY AND PORK ENTRÉES

Menu Item	Calories	Fat (g)	Sat. Fat (g)	Carbs (g)	Fiber (g)	Phase
Cajun Baked Chicken Breast (6 oz, with skin)	431	27	6	9	1	1
Grilled Chicken Breast (6 oz, with skin)	478	26	5	23	1	1
Mesquite-Smoked Chicken Breast (6 oz, without skin)	212	8	2	1	1	1
Rotisserie Chicken Breast Quarter (6 oz, with skin)	521	31	2	2	1	1
Turkey Breast (5.5 oz, without skin)	267	10	2	5	0	1
Roast Pork Loin (5 oz, bone in)	373	13	5	10	1	1

SALADS (no dressing)

Menu Item	Calories	Fat (g)	Sat. Fat (g)	Carbs (g)	Fiber (g)	Phase
Asparagus and Tomato Salad	88	5	1	10	2	1
Cauliflower Salad	117	8	2	9	2	1
Cucumber and Celery Salad	74	4	1	9	1	1
Cucumber and Tomato Salad	41	0	0	10	1	1

Menu Item	Calories	Fat (g)	Sat. Fat (g)	Carbs (g)	Fiber (g)	Phase
Cucumber Mix	61	4	1	7	2	1
Spring Salad (small)	15	0	0	3	1	1
Tomato, Cucumber, Onion Salad	44	0	0	10	1	1

SIDE DISHES

Menu Item	Calories	Fat (g)	Sat. Fat (g)	Carbs (g)	Fiber (g)	Phase
Broccoli (buttered)*	90	7	0	5	3	3
Brussels Sprouts (buttered)*	91	6	1	8	4	3
Cabbage (buttered)*	68	5	1	6	2	3
Cauliflower (buttered)*	89	6	1	8	4	3
Spinach (buttered)*	80	6	1	3	3	3

*Nutritional analysis includes butter. Request vegetables steamed to reduce fat and calories in this dish.

—⚍— Pizza Hut —⚍—

More than 6,600 restaurants nationwide
(800) 948-8488, www.pizzahut.com

With all those thousands of restaurants, it's hard not to find yourself occasionally eating at a Pizza Hut or enjoying takeout from one. In fact, Pizza Hut, which began in 1958 as a single restaurant in Wichita, Kansas, is now the world's largest pizza company. This chain is a big reason why, according to the National Association of Pizza Operators, Americans eat approximately 100 acres of pizza each day, or 350 slices per second.

BEST CHOICES

Pizza Hut's Thin 'N Crispy signature crust is the best basis for constructing a South Beach Diet–compatible pizza as an occasional treat if you're on Phase 2 or 3. Avoid the full-fat pepperoni, bacon, sausage, and beef toppings, and opt for the Veggie Lover's topping instead; it will give you a good helping of mushrooms, red onions, green peppers, tomatoes, and black olives. If you want something more substantial, order the Chicken Supreme topping, which features grilled chicken breast, green peppers, red onions, and mushrooms.

As you'll see from the nutritional analyses below, the numbers are for a single slice. If you're like most people, you may find it difficult to eat just one piece of pizza, especially when you're hungry. To help keep you from reaching for that second slice, fill out the meal with an individual tossed green salad or Caesar salad (skip the Thousand Island and French dressings). Or, if you're ordering in for the whole family or the gang at the office, ask for a Pizza Hut Bag Salad. This is a premixed salad kit that easily serves four. It contains romaine and iceberg lettuce, red cabbage, carrots, radishes, garden herb croutons, and ranch dressing—let someone else eat the croutons, and freely enjoy the rest of the salad.

RECOMMENDED DISHES

THIN 'N CRISPY PIZZA

Menu Item	Calories	Fat (g)	Sat. Fat (g)	Carbs (g)	Fiber (g)	Phase
Chicken Supreme Thin 'N Crispy Pizza (1 slice of 12-inch pizza)	200	7	3.5	22	1	2
Chicken Supreme Thin 'N Crispy Pizza (1 slice of 14-inch pizza)	180	7	3	21	1	2
Veggie Lover's Thin 'N Crispy Pizza (1 slice of 12-inch pizza)	180	7	3	23	2	2
Veggie Lover's Thin 'N Crispy Pizza (1 slice of 14-inch pizza)	170	7	3	21	2	2

—w— Planet Hollywood —w—

6 locations nationwide, 16 internationally
(407) 903-5500, www.planethollywood.com

NOTE: Nutritional information was not available for this establishment. However, we have provided some Best Choices that fit in with the South Beach Diet nutritional principles. Because we do not have specific data for these dishes, talk to your server if you have questions about the ingredients in a dish, and be especially vigilant if you are on Phase 1.

Dine with the stars—or at least their memorabilia—at one of these enjoyable theme restaurants. The Planet Hollywood chain was started in 1991 by a group of movie stars, including Bruce Willis and Sylvester Stallone. Today you can find a Planet Hollywood at six locations in major US tourist destinations, including Times Square in New York City and at Caesars Palace in Las Vegas, as well as in places like Paris, Bali, and Tokyo. All of the restaurants are decorated with an amazing collection of movie and television memorabilia from classics old and new.

BEST CHOICES

The food at Planet Hollywood is almost beside the point. There are a few things South Beach dieters can eat, however. Among the appetizers, the Oriental Lettuce Wraps are fine if you use just a dab of the dipping sauce. If you're on Phase 3, try the Southwestern Salad—grilled lime-marinated chicken, corn, black beans, mixed greens, and fontina cheese—without the tortilla strips. The Asian Chicken Salad is another interesting option. And the Grilled Chicken Caesar Salad is a good possibility for all phases if you eliminate the croutons. Among the entrées, most are off-limits, but do try the Hickory-Roasted Half Chicken (ask for extra salad instead of the potatoes).

—⁓— Qdoba Mexican Grill —⁓—

More than 200 restaurants in 30 states
(720) 898-2300, www.qdoba.com

Qdoba makes an effort to solve one of the biggest problems facing South Beach dieters: how to enjoy the authentic Mexican flavor of a burrito without the refined carbs of the tortilla wrapping. Qdoba offers the Naked Burrito—basically a tortilla-less burrito in a bowl. This menu option makes this fast-casual chain of restaurants one of the more realistic destinations for those on the South Beach Diet who love Mexican food. Even so, dieters still need to be careful.

BEST CHOICES

Any burrito on the Qdoba Mexican Grill menu, including the signature burritos, can be ordered naked. The basic Naked Burrito comes with black or pinto beans (acceptable for all phases); your choice of chicken, steak, ground sirloin, or shredded beef; lettuce, cheese, and light sour cream (also acceptable for all phases); and your choice of salsa. Unfortunately, it is served on a mound of white rice, which immediately takes it to Phase 3 status. If you ask your server to hold the rice, the burrito really does become "naked" and can be eaten by a Phase 1 dieter.

RECOMMENDED DISHES

NAKED BURRITOS AND TACOS

Menu Item	Calories	Fat (g)	Sat. Fat (g)	Carbs (g)	Fiber (g)	Phase
Naked Burrito, Chicken*	430	17	6	28	14	3
Naked Burrito, Chicken Fajita Ranchera*	450	17	6	34	14	3
Naked Burrito, Grilled Veggies*	290	10	3.5	38	15	3
Naked Taco Salad, Chicken*	370	14	6	28	8	3
Naked Taco Salad, Grilled Veggies*	240	8	3.5	33	11	3

*Nutritional analysis is for all burrito ingredients including rice. Eliminating the rice reduces the carbohydrates and calories in this dish.

—⚬— Quiznos Sub —⚬—

More than 4,000 restaurants worldwide
(866) 486-2783, www.quiznos.com

NOTE: Nutritional information was not available for this establishment. However, we have provided some Best Choices that fit in with the South Beach Diet nutritional principles. Because we do not have specific data for these dishes, talk to your server if you have questions about the ingredients in a dish, and be especially vigilant if you are on Phase 1.

When a restaurant chain has a name as unusual as Quiznos, you'd think there would be a story behind it. There isn't. The Quiznos name is invented, perhaps because Q and Z are such relatively rare letters that a name using them is instantly memorable. The chain was founded in Denver in 1981; by 1996 it had grown to 100 restaurants; by 2000 it had reached 1,000 restaurants; and in 2005 restaurant 4,000 opened. This is one of the fastest-growing food franchises in the country—if there's not one near you yet, there probably will be soon.

BEST CHOICES

Quiznos specializes in sub sandwiches served on toasted artisanal breads and topped with signature dressings, such as roasted red bell pepper. Rather than choosing one of these breads, which are high in refined carbs, request the small whole-wheat baguette. The best fillings are the roasted turkey, deli tuna, or roast beef. Ask the server to provide any sauce separately.

As an alternative to a sub, try the Roman Chicken Salad (chicken, Parmesan, Asiago, and Romano cheeses, greens, and cherry tomatoes) from the Craveable Salads list. The other large salads are too high in fat and refined carbs to be SBD-acceptable. Side Caesar and Garden salads are also available.

—~~— Rainforest Café —~~—

More than 25 restaurants in 16 states
(800) 5-LANDRY, www.rainforestcafe.com

NOTE: Nutritional information was not available for this establishment. However, we have provided some Best Choices that fit in with the South Beach Diet nutritional principles. Because we do not have specific data for these dishes, talk to your server if you have questions about the ingredients in a dish, and be especially vigilant if you are on Phase 1.

The Rainforest Café is quite literally a wild dining experience. This chain of theme restaurants features a rain forest décor with amazing animatronics, including a trumpeting elephant and a life-sized gorilla who pounds his chest in the bushes. Huge aquariums filled with colorful tropical fish add a living element to the rainforest illusion. Rainforest Cafés are family-friendly destinations found in resort areas such as Atlantic City, Las Vegas, Disneyland in California, and Disney World in Orlando.

BEST CHOICES

The menu at Rainforest Café is oriented toward family fun. While the kids might love the Congo Clam Strips appetizer served with Safari Fries, as a South Beach dieter, you shouldn't go there. In fact, from the South Beach Diet perspective, the menu is quite limited. Good choices include a Paradise House Salad or Little Islander Caesar Salad (without the croutons). As far as entrées go, the Tuscan Chicken—grilled chicken breast with cucumbers, olives, and tomatoes—is a good choice. The Shrimp Scampi Shangri-La from the seafood section of the menu is also fine—ask for extra Napa vegetables instead of rice. Another option is the Big Islander Caesar Salad with grilled chicken, grilled shrimp, or both. Again, skip the croutons.

—∾— Red Lobster —∾—

More than 670 restaurants nationwide
(800) 562-7837, www.redlobster.com

Is the restaurant chain that invented popcorn shrimp a place for a South Beach dieter to eat? Yes, because this chain also offers a good variety of seafood that's not breaded or battered and deep-fried. The chain has responded to diners looking for a healthier approach by adding the LightHouse Selections menu, which features nutritional information for each dish.

BEST CHOICES

Any sort of fish or seafood on the Red Lobster menu is not only good but good for you—as long as it's grilled, baked, blackened, roasted, or steamed, not deep-fried. That gives you a lot of options: Try the Grilled Shrimp (two skewers of garlic-grilled shrimp served with seasonal vegetables) or the LobsterChops (split Maine lobster tails wrapped around sea scallops and broiled) or the Roasted Tilapia in a Bag. That's tilapia cooked in a bag with white wine, spicy seasonings, and seasonal vegetables (you don't eat the bag). If you're not a fish or shellfish fan, the options are a lot more limited. You'll have to stick to the Grilled Chicken or the Apple Walnut Chicken Salad if you're on Phase 2. (Nutritional data was not available for these two dishes.)

Most menu items come with a side salad and seasonal vegetables; some also allow you the choice of an additional side dish. Select more vegetables, or if you're on Phase 2, try the Wild Rice Pilaf. For dishes that come with butter sauces (the Grilled Rainbow Trout or Salmon New Orleans, for instance), ask for the sauce on the side. If you do so, these dishes will become Phase 1.

continued

RECOMMENDED DISHES

FISH AND SHELLFISH ENTRÉES

Menu Item	Calories	Fat (g)	Sat. Fat (g)	Carbs (g)	Fiber (g)	Phase
Grilled Shrimp Dinner	142	3	n/a	1	0	1
Jumbo Shrimp Cocktail Dinner	228	4	n/a	2	0	1
King Crab Legs	490	9	n/a	0	0	1
LobsterChops	321	23	n/a	0	0	1
Maine Lobster	145	1	n/a	2	0	1
Roasted Tilapia in a Bag	563	16	n/a	30	10	1
Snow Crab Legs	262	5	n/a	0	0	1
Salmon New Orleans*	578	33	n/a	0	0	3
Grilled Rainbow Trout with Citrus Butter*	512	25	n/a	6	0	3

*Nutritional analysis includes butter sauce. Eliminating the butter sauce reduces fat and calories in this dish.

SIDE DISHES

Menu Item	Calories	Fat (g)	Sat. Fat (g)	Carbs (g)	Fiber (g)	Phase
Wild Rice Pilaf	204	5	n/a	36	2	2

—∾— Red Robin —∾—
Gourmet Burgers

More than 235 restaurants nationwide
(303) 846-6000, www.redrobin.com

NOTE: Nutritional information was not available for this establishment. However, we have provided some Best Choices that fit in with the South Beach Diet nutritional principles. Because we do not have specific data for these dishes, talk to your server if you have questions about the ingredients in a dish, and be especially vigilant if you are on Phase 1.

As the name says, this family-friendly chain specializes in great burgers. Founded in 1969 in Seattle, Red Robin has expanded steadily nationwide. It has a strong presence in the Pacific Northwest, California, and the Mid-Atlantic coast. Red Robin restaurants are consistent award winners for best burgers and best family-friendly establishments.

BEST CHOICES

Fortunately, Red Robin has an expansive idea of what a hamburger should be. For the best South Beach Diet choices, check the Adventuresome Burgers section of the menu. Here you'll find the Grilled Salmon Burger, the Grilled Turkey Burger, and the meatless Garden Burger—all acceptable choices as long as you ask for them bunless and have a salad instead of fries. There's also a Lettuce-Wrapped Protein Burger made with beef. Among the nonburger entrées, try the Ensenada Chicken Platter: Grilled chicken breasts are seasoned with Mexican spices and served with a side salad and two dipping sauces (skip the creamy lime sauce and go for the salsa). The Pork or Chicken Fajitas are also acceptable—just skip the tortillas (unless you're on Phase 3), and eat only the filling.

⤙ Romano's Macaroni Grill ⤚

More than 250 locations nationwide
(800) 983-4637, www.macaronigrill.com

NOTE: Nutritional information was not available for this establishment. However, we have provided some Best Choices that fit in with the South Beach Diet nutritional principles. Because we do not have specific data for these dishes, talk to your server if you have questions about the ingredients in a dish, and be especially vigilant if you are on Phase 1.

Italian food in a relaxed atmosphere is the basic concept at Romano's Macaroni Grill. Pizzas are made before your eyes in a wood-burning oven, and all the other dishes are prepared to order in the exhibition kitchen. A custom sound track of Italian music and the occasional strolling musician liven up the experience. An extensive wine cellar complements the food. If you're on Phase 2 or 3, a glass or two of wine is permissible.

BEST CHOICES

The extensive menu at a typical Romano's Macaroni Grill features more than 35 Italian specialties, all served in generous portions. Among the appetizers, those on Phase 1 should choose a small garden salad with dressing on the side. If you're on Phase 3, you can have the Mozzarella alla Caprese (mozzarella cheese, tomatoes, basil, and balsamic vinaigrette). For pasta lovers, Romano's Macaroni Grill is one of the few chains that serves whole-wheat pasta (the preferred type on the South Beach Diet)—but only in the form of penne. Try the Whole-Wheat Penne Arrabbiata (penne in a classic spicy tomato sauce) topped with grilled chicken or shrimp. The portion is large, so plan to share or take some home with you. Among the grilled items, the Chicken Portobello, the Grilled Halibut, and the Grilled Pork Chops are all fine. Other good entrées include Chicken Marsala or Veal Marsala for Phase 3 dieters. Your server will happily substitute sautéed spinach or grilled asparagus for pasta, rice, or potatoes. In the Sensible Fare section of the menu, the simple Grilled Salmon and Mediterranean Shrimp are the best options.

—✳— Rubio's Fresh —✳— Mexican Grill

More than 150 restaurants in California, Arizona,
Oregon, Colorado, Utah, and Nevada
(760) 929-8226, www.rubios.com

Rubio's Fresh Mexican Grill offers Baja-inspired specialties, including the chain's World Famous Fish Taco. This item is so popular that the chain has sold more than 50 million of them since Ralph Rubio opened his first restaurant in San Diego in 1983.

BEST CHOICES

Unfortunately, the Fish Taco isn't a good choice for a South Beach dieter—the fish is battered and deep-fried. You'll also have to stay away from all the burritos and quesadillas—they're way too high in calories, fat, and refined carbs. Some of the other taco dishes, however, are reasonable options. Even though tacos are relatively high in refined carbohydrates from the tortilla wrapping, most of the fillings are acceptable. At Rubio's, the best choice is the Chicken Street Taco—this is a smaller taco filled with grilled white meat chicken, guacamole, onions, and cilantro. If you remove the tortilla and eat only the filling, you can make a Phase 3 taco acceptable for Phase 1. For side dishes, try the Pinto Beans, Black Beans, or Guacamole. The black beans are high in fiber, and the guacamole is a good source of monounsaturated fat.

RECOMMENDED DISHES

TACOS

Menu Item	Calories	Fat (g)	Sat. Fat (g)	Carbs (g)	Fiber (g)	Phase
Chicken Street Taco (mini taco)*	110	4	0.5	10	1	3
Chicken Taco*	300	15	4	24	2	3
Healthmex Chicken Taco*	170	2	0.5	23	2	3

*Nutritional analysis includes corn tortilla. Eliminating the tortilla reduces carbohydrates, fat, and calories in this dish.

continued

SIDE DISHES

Menu Item	Calories	Fat (g)	Sat. Fat (g)	Carbs (g)	Fiber (g)	Phase
Black Beans (1 cup)	170	2	1	28	4	1
Pinto Beans (1 cup)	190	3	1.5	37	1	1
Guacamole (4 oz, small)	170	16	2.5	8	5	1

—⧓— Ruby Tuesday —⧓—

More than 700 locations in 42 states and District of Columbia
(800) 325-0755, www.rubytuesday.com

The Ruby Tuesday chain is a major player in the bar-and-grill category of casual dining. With its Smart Eating choices, the chain was also one of the first to feature healthy dishes on the menu. Look for the separate menu section and table cards that give the Smart Eating choices, along with the calories and fat, carbs, and fiber content for each dish.

BEST CHOICES

Ruby Tuesday has a fabulous salad bar with 65 different ingredients. The Famous Combo is available at any time—that's the salad bar along with garlic toast and your choice of a bowl of soup or loaded baked potato. Ask for the Smart Eating Onion Soup instead of the potato— and have it first, before you hit the salad bar. Enjoy the many assorted salad toppings and dressings by sampling them in moderate amounts atop a foundation of greens (stay away from the beets and other Phase 3 items, however).

Among the other Smart Eating options, the Burger Wraps (chicken, turkey, or veggie), which feature whole-grain tortillas, are good choices if you're on Phase 2. At any phase, the Creole Catch (broiled tilapia), Peppercorn Salmon, and Grilled Chicken are all acceptable. There's also a Skinny Chicken Salad (grilled chicken with tomatoes, cheese, and romaine lettuce with a light ranch dressing on the side) and a number of vegetable side dishes.

RECOMMENDED DISHES

SMART EATING ENTRÉES (no side dishes)

Menu Item	Calories	Fat (g)	Sat. Fat (g)	Carbs (g)	Fiber (g)	Phase
Creole Catch (tilapia)	312	16	n/a	0	0	1
Grilled Chicken	209	5	n/a	0	0	1
Peppercorn Salmon	287	15	n/a	0	0	1
Petite Sirloin	222	8	n/a	1	0	1
Top Sirloin	285	11	n/a	1	0	1
Grilled Chicken Burger Wrap*	470	24	n/a	25	10	2
Turkey Burger Wrap*	408	17	n/a	19	10	2
Veggie Burger Wrap*	449	15	n/a	42	21	2

*Nutritional analysis includes whole-grain tortilla. Eliminating the tortilla reduces carbohydrates, fat, and calories in these dishes.

SOUP, SALADS, AND SIDE DISHES

Menu Item	Calories	Fat (g)	Sat. Fat (g)	Carbs (g)	Fiber (g)	Phase
Smart Eating Onion Soup	198	13	n/a	20	0	1
Smart Eating Skinny Chicken Salad (no dressing)	283	10	n/a	13	3	1
Side Caesar Salad (no croutons)	120	10	n/a	5	1	1
Broccoli	129	8	n/a	8	3	1
Brown Rice Pilaf	223	7	n/a	36	2	2
Sugar Snap Peas	82	0	n/a	14	4	1

—∾— Ryan's —∾—
Grill, Buffet and Bakery

More than 340 restaurants in 23 states
(864) 879-1000, www.ryansrg.com

You're most likely to eat at a Ryan's Grill or its sister restaurant, Fire Mountain, if you travel the interstates in the South and Midwest. This chain has a strong presence at rest stops and near major attractions. The restaurants are family-friendly, with quick service and affordable prices.

BEST CHOICES

At Ryan's, you have the option of ordering from the menu or enjoying the Mega Bar buffet. The buffet selections vary depending on the day of the week, but on any given day you can find at least one good South Beach Diet–compatible choice, such as Grilled Chicken Breast or Baked Salmon. The buffet also gives you a chance to round out your meal with a good variety of salads and fresh vegetables.

The Ryan's menu itself offers a wider variety of entrées than the buffet. A number of healthy selections are indicated on the menu by a little smiley face symbol. In general, these are good choices for South Beach dieters and include dishes such as Grilled Pork Chops or Carved Turkey Breast. As with the buffet, the choice of vegetables and salads is fairly extensive. If you're on Phase 2 or beyond, you can select fruits such as Cantaloupe, Red Grapes, and Strawberries as a side dish option.

RECOMMENDED DISHES

ENTRÉES (all 6 oz portions)

Menu Item	Calories	Fat (g)	Sat. Fat (g)	Carbs (g)	Fiber (g)	Phase
Baked Salmon	210	10	0	0	0	1
Carved Turkey Breast	276	12	1	0	0	1
Grilled Chicken Breast	280	18	5	0	0	1
Grilled Pork Chops	240	14	5	1	0	1
Grilled Salmon	240	9	2	0	0	1

SALADS

Menu Item	Calories	Fat (g)	Sat. Fat (g)	Carbs (g)	Fiber (g)	Phase
Broccoli Cauliflower Salad with Ranch Dressing	174	12	1	8	4	1
Caesar Salad (no croutons)	174	12	1	1	1	1
Cauliflower Salad	30	0	0	6	3	1
Cucumber Salad	20	0	0	4	1	1
Greek Salad	120	12	0	4	3	1

SIDE DISHES (all 6 oz portions)

Menu Item	Calories	Fat (g)	Sat. Fat (g)	Carbs (g)	Fiber (g)	Phase
Broccoli	78	0	0	8	4	1
Brussels Sprouts	120	0	0	12	6	1
Field Peas	180	0	0	24	6	1
Green Beans	22	0	0	5	3	1
Grilled Vegetables with Broccoli	30	0	0	6	3	1
Grilled Vegetables with Cauliflower	30	0	0	6	3	1
Pinto Beans	156	1	1	24	6	1
Sautéed Mushrooms	102	1	1	8	1	1
Yellow Squash with Onions	78	0	0	10	3	1

FRUIT

Menu Item	Calories	Fat (g)	Sat. Fat (g)	Carbs (g)	Fiber (g)	Phase
Cantaloupe (1 cup)	60	0	0	13	1	2
Red Grapes (1 cup)	60	0	0	16	1	2
Strawberries (1 cup)	45	0	0	10	3	2

—⁓— Sbarro —⁓—

More than 960 restaurants worldwide
(800) 456-4837, www.sbarro.com

You'll find Sbarro restaurants mostly in shopping malls, airports, train stations, and even hospitals. This chain serves Italian food freshly prepared on the premises; the service is cafeteria-style. The open kitchen means you can watch pizzamakers spin pizza dough behind the counter. The sight is fun to see and very tempting, but unfortunately Sbarro offers only one thin-crust pizza, and many of the franchises may not yet have it listed.

BEST CHOICES

Not only must you skip the Neapolitan and Sicilian pizza offerings at Sbarro, you also need to pass up all the strombolis, calzones, and pasta dishes and most of the other entrées as well. So what *can* you fill up on? Consider the Chicken Tenders with Mixed Vegetables (fresh zucchini, yellow squash, broccoli, and baby carrots) along with one of the salad offerings, such as String Bean and Tomato.

Of course there will come the time when you're stuck in an airport and Sbarro is the most convenient place to eat. If you just can't make a meal out of chicken and vegetables, and you're on Phase 2 or beyond, you can have a slice of Thin-Crust Cheese Pizza. If you don't see it on the menu, ask for it.

RECOMMENDED DISHES

ENTRÉES AND SALADS

Menu Item	Calories	Fat (g)	Sat. Fat (g)	Carbs (g)	Fiber (g)	Phase
Thin-Crust Cheese Pizza (⅛ of a 17-inch pie)	310	14	n/a	18	0	2
Chicken Tenders with Mixed Vegetables	n/a	n/a	n/a	n/a	n/a	2
Caesar Salad (no croutons)	80	5	n/a	6	1	1
Cucumber and Tomato Salad	130	11	n/a	9	2	1

Menu Item	Calories	Fat (g)	Sat. Fat (g)	Carbs (g)	Fiber (g)	Phase
String Bean and Tomato Salad	100	7	n/a	9	2	1
Greek Salad	60	4	n/a	3	1	1
Mixed Garden Salad	35	0	n/a	0	7	1

—ᴍ— Schlotzky's Deli —ᴍ—

More than 445 restaurants in 36 states and 6 foreign countries
(800) 846-2867, www.cooldeli.com

The slogan at Schlotzky's Deli is "Funny name. Serious sandwich." Ordinarily, the sandwich part would warn South Beach dieters away from high-fat fillings and refined carb bread. At Schlotzky's, however, they're so serious about their sandwiches that they want everyone to enjoy them. You can get your sandwich the South Beach Diet way, either in a tortilla or bunless on a bed of lettuce.

BEST CHOICES

The sandwich that began it all for Schlotzky's back in 1971 in Dallas was a combination of deli meats, cheeses, and marinated black olives on sourdough bread. The Original, as it's known, is still sold at Schlotzky's, and you can now get the filling wrapped in a tortilla. That's if you're not a South Beach dieter (nearly half the calories in the Original come from fat). Look instead at the wide range of other sandwich fillings, such as Chicken Breast or Smoked Turkey Breast, and have them in a tortilla wrap (if you're on Phase 3) or breadless. If you remove the wrap, the dish moves from Phase 3 to Phase 1. Other good sandwich fillings include Dijon Chicken, Pesto Chicken, Turkey Guacamole, zesty Albacore Tuna, and Western Vegetarian.

All the leaf salads at Schlotzky's are fine for South Beach dieters. Acceptable salad dressings are traditional ranch, spicy ranch, Italian, Olde World Caesar, and Greek balsamic vinaigrette. A couple of the soups are fine as well: Vegetable Beef and Vegetarian Vegetable. Starting a meal with soup is a good way to keep from overeating.

continued

RECOMMENDED DISHES

SANDWICH FILLINGS

Menu Item	Calories	Fat (g)	Sat. Fat (g)	Carbs (g)	Fiber (g)	Phase
Albacore Tuna	334	7	n/a	2	5	1
Chicken Breast	337	3	n/a	2	5	1
Dijon Chicken	329	4	n/a	2	7	1
Pesto Chicken	346	6	n/a	2	5	1
Santa Fe Chicken	404	9	n/a	7	10	1
Smoked Turkey Breast	335	5	n/a	4	7	1
Turkey Guacamole	423	12	n/a	8	5	1
Fresh Veggie	324	7	n/a	2	7	1
Western Vegetarian	425	20	n/a	2	6	1

WRAPS

Menu Item	Calories	Fat (g)	Sat. Fat (g)	Carbs (g)	Fiber (g)	Phase
Albacore Tuna Wrap (small)*	334	7	n/a	18	9	3
Albacore Tuna and Mozzarella Toasted Wrap*	365	19	n/a	25	2	3
Dijon Chicken Wrap (small)*	329	4	n/a	14	10	3
Pesto Chicken Wrap (small)*	346	6	n/a	14	8	3
Smoked Turkey Breast Wrap (small)*	335	5	n/a	16	9	3
Turkey and Garden Vegetable Toasted Wrap*	289	9	n/a	28	3	3
Turkey Guacamole Wrap (small)*	423	12	n/a	20	11	3
Fresh Veggie Wrap (small)*	324	7	n/a	16	10	3

*Nutritional analysis includes tortilla. Eliminating the tortilla reduces carbohydrates, fat, and calories in this dish.

SOUPS AND SALADS

Menu Item	Calories	Fat (g)	Sat. Fat (g)	Carbs (g)	Fiber (g)	Phase
Vegetable Beef Soup	120	4	n/a	14	2	3
Vegetarian Vegetable Soup	138	6	n/a	20	6	3
Grilled Chicken Caesar Salad (no croutons)	169	6	n/a	11	2	1
Caesar Salad (no croutons)	101	5	n/a	10	2	1
Turkey Chef's Salad (no dressing)	261	13	n/a	12	3	1
Ham and Turkey Chef's Salad	245	13	n/a	12	4	1
Mediterranean Eggplant and Feta Salad	140	9	n/a	11	5	1
Garden Salad	50	2	n/a	8	4	1

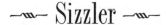

Sizzler

More than 270 restaurants in 17 states
(818) 662-9900, www.sizzler.com

The Sizzler chain began in 1957 in Culver City, California, with $50 in the cash register and four steak items on the menu. Today, this large chain of family-oriented restaurants offers a much broader menu, with many grilled items and an extensive salad bar with over 90 items.

BEST CHOICES

The Sizzler menu offers a fair number of South Beach Diet–friendly dishes. For steak lovers, the Petite Sizzler Steak, at 8 ounces, is a good choice. Other grilled choices include Hibachi Chicken and Grilled Salmon, both served with broccoli. Under the Sizzlin' Platters heading, the Garlic Herb Chicken and Grilled Shrimp Skewers are also fine (no nutritional analyses were available for these dishes). Ask for broccoli instead of potatoes, fries, or rice. You can also take advantage of the salad bar—carefully—by enjoying the greens and other veggies. But be sure to watch out for dressings with added sugar, and avoid toppings such as potato salad and crumbled bacon.

RECOMMENDED DISHES

ENTRÉES

Menu Item	Calories	Fat (g)	Sat. Fat (g)	Carbs (g)	Fiber (g)	Phase
Grilled Salmon with Broccoli	393	19	4.5	14	7	1
Hibachi Chicken with Broccoli	290	6	1	15	6	1
Petite Sizzler Steak with Broccoli (8 oz)	520	26	11	11	6	1
Sizzlin' Garlic Herb Chicken	n/a	n/a	n/a	n/a	n/a	1
Sizzlin' Grilled Shrimp Skewers	n/a	n/a	n/a	n/a	n/a	1

—ᴡ— Steak n Shake —ᴡ—

More than 430 restaurants in 19 states
(317) 633-4100, www.steaknshake.com

The venerable Steak n Shake chain dates back to 1934, when founder Gus Belt opened his first restaurant in Normal, Illinois. From the start, Gus specialized in steakburgers and milkshakes. Today the chain remains true to its roots. The Steakburger sandwich is still served, as are hand-dipped milkshakes made with real milk. In recent years, Steak n Shake has expanded the menu, which makes it just a little easier to get a good South Beach Diet–style meal.

BEST CHOICES

To start your meal and help curb your appetite, try a cup of Vegetable Beef or Chicken Gumbo Soup if you're not on Phase 1. Because the Steakburger sandwich is made with leaner beef cuts, the plain Steakburger Original Single without the bun is acceptable if you're on Phase 3. (At

Steak n Shake, your food comes on real china with real silverware, which makes that bunless option much more palatable.) Beyond the burger, your best sandwich bets are the Grilled Chicken Breast or Tuna Salad; in both cases, have them without the bun. You can also choose the Chicken Chef Salad or Deluxe Garden Salad (without the cheese) as a main course. The only side dish at Steak n Shake that's SBD-friendly is the Garden Salad. Ask for ranch dressing or oil and vinegar on the side.

RECOMMENDED DISHES

SOUPS, SALADS, AND SANDWICHES

Menu Item	Calories	Fat (g)	Sat. Fat (g)	Carbs (g)	Fiber (g)	Phase
Vegetable Beef Soup (1 cup)	117	7	2	10	2	3
Chicken Gumbo Soup (1 cup)	86	3	1	10	2	2
Chicken Chef Salad (no dressing)	463	32	12	10	3	1
Deluxe Garden Salad (no dressing)	226	15	9	10	3	1
Grilled Chicken Breast Sandwich (no bun)	246	17	3	2	0	1
Steakburger Original Single (no bun)	180	15	6	0	0	3
Tuna Salad Sandwich (no bun)	300	28	3	0	0	1
Garden Salad (no dressing)	23	0	0	5	1	1

—✺— Subway —✺—

More than 23,000 restaurants in 84 countries
(800) 888-4848, www.subway.com

South Beach dieters can put together a fine meal at Subway without too much trouble. That's good news because there are *a lot* of Subway restaurants. As one of the largest chains in America, there's almost always one in the area, no matter where you live.

BEST CHOICES

At press time, no 100 percent whole-wheat subs or wraps are available at Subway, which is why we don't recommend the sandwiches. As a South Beach dieter, you can, however, have a meal at Subway by turning any sandwich filling into a salad. Look for any good protein source, such as turkey breast, chicken breast, ham, or roast beef. Add your choice of the available vegetables: lettuce, tomato, cucumbers, onions, pickles, olives, jalapeños, and banana peppers. Dress with mayo, olive oil, or vinegar.

Subway also offers a number of prepared fresh salads such as Veggie Delite and Grilled Chicken Breast and Baby Spinach Salad. The Italian, ranch, or oil and vinegar dressings are all good choices for any of the salad offerings.

RECOMMENDED DISHES

SALADS

Menu Item	Calories	Fat (g)	Sat. Fat (g)	Carbs (g)	Fiber (g)	Phase
Chicken Breast Strips Salad	140	3	0.5	12	4	1
Grilled Chicken Breast and Baby Spinach Salad	140	3	1	11	4	1
Ham Salad	120	3	1	15	4	1
Roast Beef Salad	130	3.5	1.5	13	4	1
Subway Club Salad	160	4	1.5	15	4	1
Turkey Breast Salad	120	2.5	0.5	14	4	1
Veggie Delite Salad	60	1	0	12	4	1

—〰— Taco Bell —〰—

More than 6,500 restaurants nationwide
(800) TACO BELL, www.tacobell.com

With so many restaurants and a substantial television advertising budget, it's no surprise that Taco Bell is the largest restaurant consumer of whole iceberg lettuce in the United States. It's also not surprising that in an average year, Taco Bell uses 3.2 billion corn and flour tortillas, 260 million pounds of ground beef, and 104 million pounds of cheese.

BEST CHOICES

If you eliminate the taco salads, the gorditas, the chalupas, the burritos, and the Mexican pizzas on the grounds that they're too high in fat and refined carbs, what's left at Taco Bell are the soft tacos. Try the Soft Taco with Beef, Fresco Style, which means you can replace the cheese with Taco Bell's Fiesta Salsa (made with a mix of diced fresh tomatoes, onions, and cilantro). The Spicy Chicken Soft Taco is another good option. If you're on Phase 1 or 2, just skip the tortilla altogether and eat the filling.

Another SBD-suitable choice at Taco Bell is the Bean Burrito, which you can also order Fresco Style (again, skip the tortilla unless you're on Phase 3). This dish has 56 grams of the right carbs and lots of fiber. Another dish with good carbs is the Pintos 'n Cheese (pinto beans and cheddar cheese), which works for any phase.

RECOMMENDED DISHES

ENTRÉES AND SIDE DISHES

Menu Item	Calories	Fat (g)	Sat. Fat (g)	Carbs (g)	Fiber (g)	Phase
Soft Taco with Beef, Fresco Style*	190	8	2.5	22	2	3
Spicy Chicken Soft Taco*	180	7	2	21	2	3
Bean Burrito, Fresco Style*	350	8	2	56	9	3
Pintos 'n Cheese	180	7	3.5	20	6	1

*Nutritional analysis includes tortilla. Eliminating the tortilla reduces the carbohydrates, fat, and calories in this dish.

—∾— Taco John's —∾—

More than 400 restaurants in 27 states
(307) 635-0101, www.tacojohns.com

Taco John's is a quick-service taco restaurant in a style they call West-Mex. In addition to the usual tacos and burritos, the distinguishing offerings here are the Potato Olés—basically seasoned potato nuggets—and the Crunchy Chicken Strips. While this isn't the most South Beach Diet–friendly fast-food place around, that doesn't mean you can't eat there.

BEST CHOICES

Your best choice at Taco John's is a Chicken Soft Shell Taco or a Bean Burrito. If you're on Phase 3, you can eat the tortilla; if you're on Phase 1 or 2, simply remove it and eat the chicken or bean filling. The same is true for the Taco Burger. Remove the bun, unless you're on Phase 3. Another choice, which should be ordered only occasionally, is the Chicken Festiva Salad. It includes chargrilled chicken on lettuce with cheddar cheese, tomatoes, sour cream, and tortilla strips. Always ask your server to hold the sour cream and strips. If you're in the mood for chili, that's fine too.

RECOMMENDED DISHES

ENTRÉES

Menu Item	Calories	Fat (g)	Sat. Fat (g)	Carbs (g)	Fiber (g)	Phase
Chicken Soft Shell Taco*	190	6	3	19	4	3
Bean Burrito*	320	7	2	53	10	3
Taco Burger (no cheese)	250	9	3	28	3	3
Chili (no cheese)	210	8	3	26	4	1
Grilled Chicken Festiva Salad (no dressing)**	400	23	10	24	4	3

*Nutritional analysis includes tortilla. Eliminating the tortilla reduces carbohydrates, fat, and calories in this dish.

**Nutritional analysis includes sour cream and tortilla strips. Eliminating these reduces the carbohydrates, fat, and calories in this dish.

~~ Texas Roadhouse ~~

More than 200 restaurants in 34 states
(800) TEX-ROAD, www.texasroadhouse.com

NOTE: Nutritional information was not available for this establishment. However, we have provided some Best Choices that fit in with the South Beach Diet nutritional principles. Because we do not have specific data for these dishes, talk to your server if you have questions about the ingredients in a dish, and be especially vigilant if you are on Phase 1.

Legendary country music star Willie Nelson is one of the family at Texas Roadhouse. The restaurant chain sponsors his national concert tours, and Willie stops by the local restaurants for dinner and events as he travels across the country. The friendly, fun atmosphere at the Texas Roadhouse makes this an enjoyable place for a family dinner out—South Beach dieters included.

BEST CHOICES

The only South Beach Diet–appropriate appetizer on the menu is a cup of Texas Roadhouse Chili. Otherwise, go straight to the Hearty Steaks portion of the menu. This is one of the rare steakhouses to offer smaller steaks. The 6-ounce sirloin, along with green beans and a house salad, makes an excellent—and reasonably priced—SBD meal. Under the Country Dinners menu heading, look for the Oven-Roasted Chicken or Grilled Pork Chops. The Grilled Salmon, listed among the Dockside Favorites, is another good choice. With any of these dishes, choose a house or Caesar salad (without the croutons) and fresh vegetables as your sides. And be sure to ask your server to remove the basket of freshly baked bread that arrives when you sit down.

—∾— T.G.I. Friday's —∾—

More than 525 restaurants nationwide
(800) FRIDAYS, www.fridays.com

NOTE: Nutritional information was not available for this establishment. However, we have provided some Best Choices that fit in with the South Beach Diet nutritional principles. Because we do not have specific data for these dishes, talk to your server if you have questions about the ingredients in a dish, and be especially vigilant if you are on Phase 1.

The restaurant chain that claims it invented the term "happy hour" and brought the world Long Island iced tea began in New York City back in 1965. T.G.I. Friday's was one of the first restaurants to branch out and become a national chain. The signature Tiffany lamps and red-and-white tablecloths have recently been giving way to a more contemporary interior, but the casual, high-energy atmosphere remains.

BEST CHOICES

The menu at T.G.I. Friday's is extensive, and South Beach dieters will have to read it carefully to find good choices. Skip the appetizers and look to the salads. Both the Santa Fe Chicken Salad (without the corn salsa) and the Grilled Chicken Caesar Salad (without the croutons) are fine as a main course. Other entrée possibilities include Chargrilled Salmon or Chargrilled Chicken Breasts. You can also have the Bruschetta Grouper, a mild white fish topped with tomatoes, or the 10-ounce Classic Sirloin (take some home). Order extra broccoli in place of the white rice. The Chicken Fajitas and Steak Fajitas are also possibilities since they don't come with tortillas but rather in a skillet full of roasted onions and red and green peppers.

—⚬— Tony Roma's —⚬—

More than 115 restaurants in 26 states
(214) 343-7800, www.tonyromas.com

NOTE: Nutritional information was not available for this establishment. However, we have provided some Best Choices that fit in with the South Beach Diet nutritional principles. Because we do not have specific data for these dishes, talk to your server if you have questions about the ingredients in a dish, and be especially vigilant if you are on Phase 1.

The original Tony Roma's was a hamburger restaurant in North Miami, Florida. Tony made his place famous for ribs in 1972, when he started serving baby back ribs from the grill. The chain now has over 260 restaurants in 27 countries and has won numerous awards over the years for its ribs and signature sauces.

BEST CHOICES

Barbecued ribs are off-limits for South Beach dieters—the sauce usually contains added sugar, and ribs are high in saturated fat. Since you can't have ribs, there are other options. The Marinated Chicken Grill, Grilled Gulf Shrimp Skewers, and Tony's 8-ounce Sirloin are all good South Beach Diet choices. Other possibilities include the Grilled Chicken Caesar Salad, Grilled Chicken Salad (hold the tortilla strips), and Tony's Asian Salad (hold the fried wonton noodles). The side dishes are limited—ask for fresh vegetables or the Roma Tomato Pesto Salad.

—ᴡᴡ— Uno Chicago Grill —ᴡᴡ—

More than 200 restaurants in 32 states
(617) 323-9200, www.unos.com

You might remember this restaurant chain from when it was called Pizzeria Uno. The chain has its roots in Chicago back in 1943, where Ike Sewell invented deep-dish pizza, a style that became so associated with his city that it's sometimes called Chicago pizza. When Ike opened Pizzeria Uno and began serving his invention, the restaurant rapidly became so popular that he needed to expand. At the first pizzeria, however, there wasn't any room, so Ike opened Pizzeria Due across the street on the lower level of a beautiful old Victorian mansion. The two pizzerias have since become world-famous Chicago fixtures.

BEST CHOICES

Deep-dish pizza is still the featured menu item at Uno Chicago Grill, and it's not for South Beach dieters. But today the franchised restaurants also offer a broader choice. For example, the so-called Topped Salads at Uno Chicago Grill—in which a House or Caesar Salad is topped off with your choice of Grilled Chicken, Roasted Turkey Breast, or Grilled Shrimp—are all fine. These go from Phase 3 to Phase 1 if you hold the croutons and have the dressing on the side. Other good options include dishes like Grilled Chicken Breast and Lemon Basil Salmon. Choose Broccoli Florets, a combo of Steamed or Roasted Vegetables, or Coleslaw as side dishes.

RECOMMENDED DISHES

SALADS (with dressing)

Menu Item	Calories	Fat (g)	Sat. Fat (g)	Carbs (g)	Fiber (g)	Phase
House Salad	120	1	0	25	5	3
Grilled Chicken House Salad (with croutons)*	350	10	1	25	5	3
Grilled Shrimp House Salad (with croutons)*	280	12	2	27	6	3

Menu Item	Calories	Fat (g)	Sat. Fat (g)	Carbs (g)	Fiber (g)	Phase
Turkey House Salad (with croutons)*	290	12	3	25	5	**3**
Gorgonzola Walnut Salad (with croutons)*	200	13	4	17	4	**3**
Tomato, Mozzarella, Basil Salad	160	13	5	3	1	**3**
Caesar Salad (with croutons)*	430	37	9	21	5	**3**

*Nutritional analysis includes croutons. Eliminating the croutons reduces carbohydrates, fat, and calories in this dish.

ENTRÉES

Menu Item	Calories	Fat (g)	Sat. Fat (g)	Carbs (g)	Fiber (g)	Phase
Grilled Chicken Breast	240	9	0.5	0	0	**1**
Lemon Basil Salmon	480	38	7	0	0	**1**

SIDE DISHES

Menu Item	Calories	Fat (g)	Sat. Fat (g)	Carbs (g)	Fiber (g)	Phase
Broccoli Florets	110	10	2	5	3	**1**
Coleslaw	120	7	1	13	1	**2**
Roasted Veggies	100	5	1	13	3	**2**
Seasoned Steamed Veggies	60	2	0	9	3	**1**

—⚜— Wendy's —⚜—

More than 6,000 locations nationwide
(614) 764-3100, www.wendys.com

The official name of this immensely popular fast-food chain is Wendy's Old-Fashioned Hamburgers. Even so, it's still possible to get a reasonable South Beach Diet meal at a Wendy's franchise. Grilled Chicken has been on the menu at Wendy's since 1983, and fresh salads have been an option since 1992.

BEST CHOICES

To enjoy an Old-Fashioned Hamburger at Wendy's, choose the Classic Single—hold the bun and ketchup, but enjoy the pickles, lettuce, onion, and tomato. Even without the bun and accompaniments, the burger remains a Phase 3 dish because of our concern about saturated fat. The Ultimate Chicken Grill Sandwich is a better choice as long as you toss the bun. Stay away from the chicken strips and nuggets—they're breaded and fried. If you'd like a little variety, try a small cup of Chili along with a side salad. The best choices at Wendy's, however, are the Garden Sensation Salads—as long as you toss any bacon pieces and croutons and have the ranch or Caesar dressing on the side. You can eat everything that comes with the Mediterranean Chicken Salad, but use the ranch or Caesar sparingly.

RECOMMENDED DISHES

SANDWICHES

Menu Item	Calories	Fat (g)	Sat. Fat (g)	Carbs (g)	Fiber (g)	Phase
Classic Single Hamburger (no bun, no ketchup)	260	18	6	4	1	3
Ultimate Chicken Grill Sandwich (no bun)	160	4.5	1	6	1	1

SALADS (no dressing)

Menu Item	Calories	Fat (g)	Sat. Fat (g)	Carbs (g)	Fiber (g)	Phase
Garden Sensation Chicken BLT Salad (no croutons)*	340	18	9	12	4	3
Garden Sensation Mediterranean Chicken Salad	280	12	7	14	5	1
Garden Sensation Mandarin Chicken Salad	170	2	0.5	18	3	2
Spring Mix Salad (with cheddar and Jack cheese)	180	11	6	13	4	1
Caesar Side Salad (no croutons)	70	5	2	3	2	1
Side Salad	35	0	0	8	2	1

*Nutritional analysis includes bacon. Eliminating the bacon reduces carbohydrates, fat, and calories in this dish.

OTHER ITEMS

Menu Item	Calories	Fat (g)	Sat. Fat (g)	Carbs (g)	Fiber (g)	Phase
Chili (small, no cheese)	220	6	2.5	23	5	3
Fresh Fruit Cup	130	5	1	33	3	3

∼∼ Whataburger ∼∼

More than 575 restaurants nationwide
(361) 878-0650, www.whataburger.com

When he founded his first restaurant in 1950 in south Texas, Harmon Dobson wanted to serve his customers something that would make them exclaim, "What a burger!" He succeeded, and soon the familiar orange-and-white-striped A-frame structures that are the Whataburger trademark began to dot the South and then other parts of the country. Whataburgers are still primarily family-friendly hamburger restaurants, but the chain does offer a few items that are also fine for South Beach Dieters.

BEST CHOICES

Whataburger restaurants are very cooperative about customizing your meal. That basically means you can get a bunless Whataburger or a bunless Grilled Chicken Sandwich. Of the two, the better choice is the chicken, but then again, it's hard not to eat a burger at Whataburger. We've assigned it to Phase 3, even without the bun, because of our concern about saturated fat. The only other real option is the Grilled Chicken Salad—stick to the ranch or Caesar dressing.

RECOMMENDED DISHES

ENTRÉES AND SIDE DISHES

Menu Item	Calories	Fat (g)	Sat. Fat (g)	Carbs (g)	Fiber (g)	Phase
Whataburger (no bun)	270	18	n/a	4	1	3
Grilled Chicken Salad (no dressing)	229	7	n/a	19	5	1
Grilled Chicken Sandwich (no bun)	190	7	n/a	10	1	1
Garden Salad (no dressing)	48	0	0	10	4	1

BUSINESS
DINING

In this section, we've selected some of the top restaurants for business dining in 15 major American cities. Whether you're traveling for work or entertaining clients or guests in your hometown, these restaurants make dining out a pleasure for South Beach dieters. In every city, we suggest places with outstanding food, excellent service, and a pleasant atmosphere. Often these are locally owned restaurants, but sometimes we've included popular destinations like Morton's with branches in a number of cities included in this guide (in such cases we've listed those cities).

For each restaurant, we've provided a brief description of the cuisine and ambience and selected the most South Beach Diet–friendly dishes from a typical menu. Remember that the menus at fine restaurants change often depending on the season and what's freshest in the market. If you don't find a particular dish we've mentioned, there's probably something similar available.

To help you stay on track, we've taken the liberty of listing menu items without the starches or rich sauces and dressings that are often part of the presentation (and that you need to ask your server to leave off your plate). That's why you'll see so many dishes marked All Phases. If you see an item labeled Phase 2 or 3, it's because of our concern about the saturated fat in the cheese, sauce, or dressing in the dish. When ordering, ask for dressings and sauces on the side; replace the bread, potatoes, rice, and other starches with extra vegetables; and choose grilled items instead of fried foods. Also ask if the chef can prepare your vegetables in olive oil or as little butter as possible. The staff at a fine restaurant wants you to enjoy your meal and will do all they can to accommodate you.

❧ Chops and the Lobster Bar ❧

70 West Paces Ferry Road, Atlanta, GA 30305
(404) 262-2675, www.buckheadrestaurants.com

Consistently ranked as one of the top steakhouses not just in Atlanta but in the United States, Chops is really two separate settings sharing one fabulous kitchen. The upper level is an intimate steakhouse dining room decorated in dark woods and palms; an elevator ride down is the Lobster Bar, with arched ceilings covered in white tile and offering fresh seafood (the same menu applies). Either dining room is a good place for South Beach dieters, though the steakhouse is perhaps better for a business meal. Many of the dishes come with potatoes or rice, so ask for steamed vegetables instead.

APPETIZERS AND SALADS

Smoked Atlantic Salmon	ALL PHASES
Classic Steak Tartare	ALL PHASES
Jumbo Lump Crab Cocktail	ALL PHASES
Chops "Chopped Salad"	ALL PHASES

ENTRÉES

Prime New York Strip (12 oz)	ALL PHASES
Center Cut Filet Mignon (8 oz)	ALL PHASES
Domestic Loin Lamb Chops, Triple Cut	ALL PHASES
Seared Atlantic Salmon with Wilted Spinach	ALL PHASES
Cracked Pepper Ahi Tuna Steak with Shiitakes	ALL PHASES
Chilean Sea Bass with Spinach	ALL PHASES
Horseradish-Crusted Atlantic Grouper	ALL PHASES
Sautéed Whole Dover Sole	ALL PHASES

SIDE DISHES

Little Joe's Spinach and Mushrooms	ALL PHASES
Fresh Steamed Broccoli	ALL PHASES
Fresh Green Beans Sautéed	ALL PHASES

❧ Kyma ☙

3085 Piedmont Road, Atlanta, GA 30305
(404) 262-0702, www.buckheadrestaurants.com

Greek cuisine is the hallmark of this contemporary version of a seafood tavern. The dramatic design offers bold white marble columns, a waterfall fountain cascading to a display of iced fresh fish, and a deep-blue ceiling adorned with twinkling constellations. Begin your meal here with a selection of mezedes, or Greek appetizers. Then move on to the house specialty, wood-grilled seafood (just be sure to substitute one of the side dishes recommended below for the popular Greek-style potatoes).

APPETIZERS, SOUPS, AND SALADS

Grilled Red and Yellow Holland Sweet Peppers with White Anchovies	ALL PHASES
Wood-Grilled Octopus with Red Onions	ALL PHASES
Greek Fisherman's Soup	ALL PHASES
Baked Whole Prawns with Tomatoes and Feta	PHASE 2
Spinach and Cheese–Stuffed Grilled Maine Calamari	PHASE 3

ENTRÉES

Wood-Grilled Royal Dorado	ALL PHASES
Wood-Grilled Red Snapper	ALL PHASES
Wood-Grilled Whole Prawns	ALL PHASES
Pan-Sautéed Dover Sole	ALL PHASES
Grilled Swordfish with Onions, Peppers, and Tomatoes	ALL PHASES
Single-Cut Lamb Chops	ALL PHASES

SIDE DISHES

Slow-Cooked Eggplant Stew	ALL PHASES
Wilted Wild Greens	ALL PHASES
Chilled Thin Beans	ALL PHASES
Giant White Kastorian Beans	ALL PHASES

❧ Rathbun's ☙

112 Krog Street, Suite R, Atlanta, Georgia 30307
(404) 524-8280, www.rathbunsrestaurant.com

After years of training in fine kitchens around the country, executive chef Kevin Rathbun opened his own restaurant in 2004. The menu is eclectic, offering, as the chef says, "seasonally and globally driven food." Located in the hip Inman Park area, Rathbun's is in a renovated industrial site that was formerly a stove factory. The main dining room is a bit on the noisy side—for a quieter evening, choose the patio.

APPETIZERS AND SALADS

Thai Rare Beef and Red Onion Salad	ALL PHASES
Georgia Shrimp with Spicy Chile Garlic Sauce	ALL PHASES
Ahi Tuna "Crudo" with Cold-Pressed Olive Oil	ALL PHASES
Hamachi, Chilled Dashi, Cucumber, and Sesame	ALL PHASES
Thin and Raw Beef Sirloin	ALL PHASES
Georgia Zucchini and Parmesan Reggiano Salad	ALL PHASES
Local Field Greens with Shaved Manchego	ALL PHASES
Romaine Heart Salad with Gruyère Cheese	PHASE 2
Monkfish Piccata with Crisp Capers	PHASE 3
Mozzarella with Sun-Dried Tomatoes and Organic Capers	PHASE 3

ENTRÉES

Seared Yellow Fin Tuna	ALL PHASES
Rosemary Grilled Beef Flat Iron Steak	ALL PHASES
Kobe Beef Culotte with Red Pepper Chimichurri	ALL PHASES

SIDE DISHES

Sautéed Garlic Spinach with Tuscan Olive Oil	ALL PHASES
Stem-On Grilled Artichokes with First-Press Olive Oil	ALL PHASES

❧ South City Kitchen ☙

1144 Crescent Avenue, Atlanta, GA 30309
(404) 873-7358, www.southcitykitchen.com

Specializing in contemporary Southern cuisine, South City Kitchen serves a sophisticated blend of Low Country Southern favorites and newer flavors. The restaurant combines the energy of the big city with down-home Southern warmth. South City Kitchen is in a renovated frame house with a large dining patio, which only adds to the homey feel. The locale, however, is bustling midtown Atlanta, close to many performance venues.

APPETIZERS AND SALADS

Pickled Gulf Shrimp Cocktail	ALL PHASES
Caesar Salad with Calabash Shrimp	ALL PHASES
Heirloom Tomato Salad with Shaved Red Onions	ALL PHASES
Mixed Field Greens with Julienne Vegetables	ALL PHASES
Seared Sea Scallops with Watermelon-Shaved Fennel Salad	PHASE 3

ENTRÉES

Roast Vegetable Napoleon	ALL PHASES
Grilled Tuna Steak with Roasted Pepper-Artichoke Salad	ALL PHASES
Pork Chop Stuffed with Tomato and Asiago Cheese	PHASE 2
Oven-Roasted Salmon with Pickled Okra Salad	PHASE 3
Pan-Roasted Georgia Trout with Truffled Creamed Corn	PHASE 3

SIDE DISHES

Asparagus	ALL PHASES
Thin Green Beans	ALL PHASES
Swiss Chard	ALL PHASES
Collard Greens	PHASE 2

❦ Veni Vidi Vici ❦

41 14th Street, Atlanta, GA 30309
(404) 875-8424, www.buckheadrestaurants.com

Simple, straightforward Italian cooking makes Veni Vidi Vici (VVV to its fans) a favorite for diners in midtown Atlanta. Close to many cultural venues, VVV is a good choice for a pretheater meal or business dinner. Grilled meats and fish prepared on an open wood–fired rotisserie are a specialty at VVV, making this restaurant ideal for South Beach dieters who enjoy Italian food.

APPETIZERS AND SALADS

Grilled Octopus	ALL PHASES
Roasted Red and Yellow Peppers	ALL PHASES
Grilled Roman-Style Artichoke	ALL PHASES
Green Salad with Balsamic Vinaigrette	ALL PHASES
Roasted Portobellos and Arugula	ALL PHASES
Thin-Sliced Air-Dried Beef	ALL PHASES
Buffalo Mozzarella with Ripe Summer Tomatoes	PHASE 3

ENTRÉES

Chicken with Broccoli Rabe	ALL PHASES
Grilled Salmon with Cannellini Beans	ALL PHASES
Grilled Veal Chop	ALL PHASES
Seafood Soup in Tomato Saffron Broth	ALL PHASES
Grilled Lamb Chops "Scottaditi" with Roasted Beets	PHASE 3

SIDE DISHES

Grilled Asparagus with Shaved Pecorino	ALL PHASES
Garlicky Thin Green Beans	ALL PHASES
Sautéed Spinach with Parmigiano Crumbs	ALL PHASES

❧ Blackfin Chop ☙
House & Raw Bar

116 Huntington Avenue, Boston, MA 02116
(617) 247-2400, www.blackfinchophouse.com

Blackfin features seafood, dry-aged meats, and a custom-built raw bar, all in a landmark Back Bay location. The cuisine here is adventurous contemporary American. The seafood is impressively fresh and varied, reflecting the strong affinity owner/chef Anthony Ambrose feels for the ocean. The raw bar offers only the freshest shellfish and seafood—most of it is purchased directly from local fishermen. Back in the kitchen, fish is cooked using grapeseed oil, a light oil that allows its flavor to come through. Seafood entrées are served with seasonal vegetables; ask for vegetables instead of potatoes with the meat entrées.

APPETIZERS AND SALADS

Steamed Mussels with Spicy Tomato Broth	ALL PHASES
Oysters on the Half Shell	ALL PHASES
Jonah Crab Claws with Dijon Sauce	ALL PHASES
Jumbo Shrimp Cocktail with Horseradish Sauce	ALL PHASES
Tuna Tartare with Tomatoes, Capers, and Spring Onions	ALL PHASES

ENTREÉS

New England Fish Pier Daily Selections	ALL PHASES
Filet Mignon (12 oz)	ALL PHASES
Pan-Roasted Monkfish Loin	ALL PHASES
Swordfish Grilled over Wood with Scallop Hash	PHASE 2

SIDE DISHES

Sautéed Asparagus	ALL PHASES
Sautéed Seasonal Vegetables	ALL PHASES
Whipped Sweet Potatoes	PHASE 3

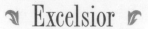 Excelsior

The Heritage on the Garden
272 Boylston Street, Boston, MA 02116
(617) 426-7878, www.excelsiorrestaurant.com

Entering Excelsior is dramatic—diners come in through the sleek first-floor bar, then take an all-glass elevator through the amazing three-story wine tower to the exquisite dining room overlooking Boston's Public Garden. After that sort of buildup, the food needs to be extraordinary, and it is. The chef's cooking is innovative yet uncomplicated, with the fundamental flavors of ingredients the focus of each dish. The restaurant is happy to adapt dishes such as the Grand Vegetable Platter to accommodate South Beach dieters on any phase.

APPETIZERS, SOUPS, AND SALADS

Seared Steak Tartare "Au Poivre"	ALL PHASES
Blue Crab and Red Lentil Soup	ALL PHASES
"Hard Cider" Cured Arctic Char Gravlax	PHASE 2
Excelsior Caesar Salad with Moullard Duck Prosciutto	PHASE 3

ENTRÉES

Grilled Prime Sirloin Steak	ALL PHASES
Day Boat Cod in Toasted Shallot Crust	PHASE 2
Grilled Lamb Rack and Lamb Shoulder Confit	PHASE 2

SIDE DISHES

Asparagus Spears	ALL PHASES
Sautéed Spinach	ALL PHASES
Grand Vegetable Platter	ALL PHASES
Mushrooms with Amontillado Sherry	PHASE 2

❧ Mistral ☙

223 Columbus Avenue, Boston, MA 02116
(617) 867-9300, www.mistralbistro.com

Mistral is located in Boston's trendy South End. The dramatic, candlelit dining room is decorated with traditional Provençal materials—stucco, stone, iron, and wood adorn the high ceilings and arched, floor-to-ceiling windows. Since its opening in 1997, Mistral has received accolades in numerous publications, including *Esquire, Fortune,* and *Food & Wine.* The food at this popular restaurant is simple, robust, and consistently excellent, the wine list is outstanding, and the service is highly professional. South Beach dieters dining here for business or pleasure should skip the potatoes, risotto, semolina toasts, and crispy wontons that come with some dishes.

APPETIZERS AND SALADS

Grilled Portobello Mushroom "Carpaccio"	ALL PHASES
Steamed Black Mussels with Smoked Tomato Marinière	ALL PHASES
Sushi-Grade Tuna Tartare	ALL PHASES
Lamb's Lettuce with Soft Goat Cheese and Pecan Melba	PHASE 3

ENTRÉES

Roasted Cornish Game Hen	ALL PHASES
Pan-Roasted Halibut	ALL PHASES
Dover Sole Meunière	PHASE 3
Roast Rack of Lamb with Celery Root Gratin	PHASE 3
Grilled Atlantic Salmon with Fall Vegetable Roti	PHASE 3
Skillet-Roasted Prime Sirloin "Au Poivre"	PHASE 3

❧ No. 9 Park ❧

Nine Park Street, Boston, MA 02108
(617) 742-9991, www.no9park.com

Soon after No. 9 Park opened in 1998, it was named one of the top new restaurants in America by *Bon Appétit* magazine. It's easy to see why. Located in an elegant townhouse in Boston's historic Beacon Hill, No. 9 Park serves regionally inspired Italian and French dishes with an emphasis on simplicity and flavor. There's also a fine wine list. The chef uses artisanal ingredients whenever possible and adjusts the menus often to reflect the changing seasons. If you're on Phase 1, ask your server about substituting steamed vegetables for some of the more complicated side dishes in the menu items marked Phase 2 or 3, below.

APPETIZERS AND SALADS

Oysters on the Half Shell with Mignonette	ALL PHASES
Aubergine Gratin with Tomato Confit and Swiss Chard Emulsion	PHASE 3
Assiette of Baby Beets with Toasted Pistachios and Chèvre	PHASE 3

ENTRÉES

Seared Rosefish with Saffron-Braised Endive	ALL PHASES
Tasting of Lamb with Oven-Dried Tomatoes	ALL PHASES
Coriander-Crusted Monkfish with Carrot and Ginger Purée	PHASE 2
Colorado Lamb with Vidalia Onion Fondue	PHASE 2
Sous Vide Suckling Pig	PHASE 3
Duet of Pheasant with Fall Vegetables	PHASE 3

❧ Radius ☙

Eight High Street, Boston, MA 02110
(617) 426-1234, www.radiusrestaurant.com

The modern French menu at Radius is a lighter version of classic French cuisine. It's marked by an emphasis on seasonal ingredients, classical technique, and the use of flavored oils, emulsions, juices, and reductions. The menu here changes often, depending on the season, the market, and what catches the chef's attention. No matter what you order, it's served with consummate professionalism in the dramatic circular dining room. Radius also has upstairs and downstairs lounges suitable for quiet conversation and rooms that can be booked for private dining.

APPETIZERS, SOUPS, AND SALADS

Chilled Pea Soup with Poached Shrimp and Mint	ALL PHASES
Vermont Rabbit Salad with Roasted Cèpes and Arugula	ALL PHASES
Spicy Shrimp Salad with Red Chiles	ALL PHASES
Sashimi of Ahi Tuna with Avocado and Orange	PHASE 2

ENTREÉS

Herb-Basted Giannone Chicken with Black Trumpet Mushrooms	ALL PHASES
Seared Chatham Cod with Zucchini and Piquillo Peppers	ALL PHASES
Vegetables 5 Ways	ALL PHASES
Duo of Colorado Lamb with Broccoli Rabe, Shallots, and Cumin Juice	ALL PHASES
Virginia Black Bass with Roasted Cauliflower and Apple Salad	PHASE 2
Scottish Salmon with Spinach, Beets, and Caviar Sauce	PHASE 3

❧ Japonais ❧

600 West Chicago Avenue, Chicago, IL 60610
(312) 822-9600, www.japonaischicago.com

Modern-day Japan meets European elegance in this sophisticated restaurant. The carefully prepared food is beautifully presented and served. Traditional Japanese dishes are available, including an outstanding choice of sushi and sashimi (stick with sashimi if you're on Phase 1 or 2), but you're better off sampling the entrées for an entirely new perspective on Japanese cuisine. Stay away from the Satsumaimo Pommes (fried sweet potatoes), and ask for sauces on the side. Unfortunately, the extensive sake list is also off-limits for South Beach dieters.

APPETIZERS, SOUPS, AND SALADS

Marinated Sashimi Baby Tuna	ALL PHASES
Kobe Beef Carpaccio	ALL PHASES
Miso Soup	ALL PHASES
Thinly Sliced Marinated New York Strip Steak Cooked on a Hot Rock	ALL PHASES
Marinated Sweet Vinegar Seaweed Salad with Toasted Sesame and Fresh Cucumbers	PHASE 3

ENTRÉES

Samurai-Cut Tuna Steak with Wasabe Glaze	ALL PHASES
Filet Mignon (8 oz) with Asparagus	ALL PHASES
Sake and Mirin Broiled Lobster with Grilled Filet Mignon and Broccolini	PHASE 3
Kobe Beef Prime Rib	PHASE 3

SIDE DISHES

Sesame Asparagus	ALL PHASES
Steamed Broccolini	ALL PHASES

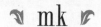 mk

868 North Franklin Street, Chicago, IL 60610
(312) 482-9179, www.mkchicago.com

Celebrated chef Michael Kornick is the man behind the name of this popular restaurant, located in Chicago's River North gallery district. Chef Kornick's adventuresome cooking is a blend of traditional French and contemporary American, and he prefers to utilize the freshest ingredients from local green markets. The stylish cuisine at mk is a perfect match for the chic two-tiered dining area, which appears to hang from the rafters and features angled skylights.

APPETIZERS AND SALADS

Chilled Oysters on the Half Shell	ALL PHASES
Baby Octopus with Grilled Frisée	ALL PHASES
Grilled Prince Edward Island Mussels	ALL PHASES
Baby Arugula with Goat Cheese	ALL PHASES
Golden Tomato Gazpacho with Peekytoe Crab	ALL PHASES
Salad of Belgian Endive with Apple and Toasted Pecans	PHASE 2
Chilled Maine Lobster with Nectarines and Fennel	PHASE 2

ENTRÉES

Atlantic Salmon with Shiitake Mushrooms	ALL PHASES
Pan-Roasted Alaskan Halibut with Braised Leeks	ALL PHASES
Roasted Loin of Lamb with Cucumber and Mint-Scented Yogurt	ALL PHASES
Seared California Yellowtail with Sugar Snap Peas	ALL PHASES
Roasted Berkshire Pork Rib Chop with Heirloom Tomato Panzanella	PHASE 3

❧ Morton's ❧

1050 North State Street, Chicago, IL 60610
(312) 266-4820, www.mortons.com

Morton's steakhouse restaurants are found in a number of major cities, but this location north of downtown Chicago is the flagship. Morton's is a genuine steakhouse, with a clubby atmosphere and very generous portions. The restaurant prides itself on cooking its steaks at 1,200 degrees to "seal in the juicy goodness." For appetizers and salads, South Beach dieters should ask for a half portion and avoid the dressings and croutons. For steaks, select the leaner cuts, such as New York strip or filet mignon, and remember that even Morton's "Slightly Smaller" steaks are still 14 ounces. Be sure to have your server hold the creamy béarnaise and au poivre sauces.

APPETIZERS AND SALADS

Jumbo Lump Crabmeat Cocktail	ALL PHASES
Colossal Shrimp Cocktail	ALL PHASES
Grilled Asparagus	ALL PHASES
Morton's Salad (romaine, chopped egg, anchovies)	ALL PHASES
Caesar Salad (no croutons)	ALL PHASES

ENTRÉES

New York Strip Steak (14 oz)	ALL PHASES
Single Cut Filet Mignon (14 oz)	ALL PHASES
Domestic Double Rib Lamb Chops (6 oz each)	ALL PHASES
Whole Baked Maine Lobster	ALL PHASES

SIDE DISHES

Steamed Fresh Asparagus	ALL PHASES
Steamed Fresh Broccoli	ALL PHASES
Sautéed Fresh Spinach and Mushrooms	ALL PHASES
Sautéed Wild Mushrooms	ALL PHASES

★ *You can find a Morton's in every city featured in this dining guide.*

❧ The Signature Room ☙ at the 95th

875 North Michigan Avenue, Chicago, IL 60611
(312) 787-9596, www.signatureroom.com

Located on the 95th floor of the John Hancock Center, one of the tallest buildings in Chicago, The Signature Room provides unequaled views of the city and Lake Michigan. Its slogan is: "The restaurant Chicago looks up to." The food—straightforward contemporary American with European and Asian influences—is a match for the view. This restaurant is a popular place for marriage proposals, but the upscale casual atmosphere makes it a good choice for business dining as well.

APPETIZERS AND SALADS

Seared Ahi Tuna with Sichuan Peppercorn Crust	ALL PHASES
Warm Marinated Gulf Shrimp with Roasted Garlic Purée	ALL PHASES
Farmer's Market Mixed Greens	ALL PHASES
Signature Caesar Salad (no croutons)	ALL PHASES

ENTRÉES

Organic Breast of Chicken	ALL PHASES
Sautéed American Red Snapper with Japanese Eggplant	ALL PHASES
Slow-Roasted Rack of Lamb with Haricot Vert	ALL PHASES
Grilled Pork Porterhouse with Sun-Dried Cherry Sauce	PHASE 2
Crispy Filet of Wild King Salmon in Pinot Noir Sauce	PHASE 3

SIDE DISHES

Steamed Asparagus Spears	ALL PHASES
Seasonal Vegetables	ALL PHASES

❦ Spiaggia ❧

980 North Michigan Avenue, Level 2, Chicago, IL 60611
(312) 280-2750, www.levyrestaurants.com

With its original décor and award-winning cuisine, Spiaggia is one of the finest Italian dining experiences in Chicago—and perhaps the entire Midwest. The 40-foot windows in this opulent restaurant look out on magnificent views of Lake Michigan. Custom-designed Italian chandeliers provide gentle lighting, and booths set between black marble pillars offer privacy for business diners. Outstanding service and an excellent wine cellar complement the imaginative menu. Skip the pasta and look for the South Beach–friendly seafood dishes that really set Spiaggia apart.

APPETIZERS AND SALADS

Wood-Roasted Sea Scallops with Porcini Mushrooms and Parmigiano-Reggiano	ALL PHASES
Organic Salmon with Lemon and Arugula	ALL PHASES
Langostinos with Green Beans	ALL PHASES
Arugula with Shaved Pressed Ricotta Cheese	ALL PHASES

ENTRÉES

Wood-Roasted Turbot	ALL PHASES
Wood-Roasted Mediterranean Sea Bass	ALL PHASES
Wood-Grilled Dorade Royale with Artichoke Purée	ALL PHASES
Olive Oil–Poached Lobster with Baby Zucchini and Osetra Caviar	ALL PHASES
Wood-Roasted Heirloom Berkshire Pork Loin with Braised Tuscan Greens and Grilled Figs	PHASE 2

❧ Blue Point Grille ☙

700 West St. Clair Avenue, Cleveland, OH 44113
(216) 875-7827, www.hrcleveland.com

A fine seafood restaurant near the shores of Lake Erie might seem a contradiction in terms, but the resourceful buyers at Blue Point Grille manage to find the freshest fish and shellfish from around the country and the world. Oysters are the signature dish here—some 75,000 of them get eaten by diners at Blue Point Grille every year. Other house specialties include a number of good South Beach Diet–compatible options. Look for the section of the menu titled "Simply Prepared" to find the best choices.

APPETIZERS AND SALADS

Shrimp Cocktail	ALL PHASES
Steamed P.E.I. Mussels in Roma Tomato Broth	ALL PHASES
Chilled Long Island Blue Point Oysters on the Half Shell	ALL PHASES
Seared Tuna with Fresh Oregon Wasabi and Seaweed Carrot Slaw	PHASE 2

ENTRÉES

Seared Singapore Tuna with Sautéed Asian Greens	ALL PHASES
Banana Leaf–Wrapped Halibut with Lemon Grass, Cucumbers, and Yogurt	ALL PHASES
Sautéed Carolina Black Grouper	ALL PHASES
Pacific Swordfish with Rock Shrimp and Tomatilla Salsa	ALL PHASES
Seared Sea Scallops with Vegetable Sauté and Pecan Vinaigrette	ALL PHASES
Oven-Roasted Chicken with Asparagus	ALL PHASES
Center Cut Filet Mignon (8 oz)	ALL PHASES

❧ Johnny's Downtown ☙

1406 West 6th Street, Cleveland, OH 44113
(216) 623-0055

The funky Warehouse District of downtown Cleveland is the city's bustling new restaurant area. One of the hot spots is Johnny's Downtown (a relative of the venerable Johnny's Bar on the Near West Side). Here visiting celebrities and sports stars can often be spotted dining on the excellent Italian/Continental cuisine. From the South Beach Diet perspective, the many pasta dishes (not allowed on Phase 1 and very limited on Phase 2 and 3) are balanced by a good selection of seafood dishes. Because the fish and shellfish menu changes regularly depending on what's available and freshest that day, ask your server for the best options.

APPETIZERS AND SALADS

House-Cured Gravlax	ALL PHASES
Mustard Seed and Coriander Seared Tuna Sashimi	ALL PHASES
Grilled Shrimp and Greek White Bean Salad with Baby Tomatoes and Shaved Asiago	ALL PHASES
Mozzarella Marinara	PHASE 3

ENTRÉES

Fresh Fish of the Day	ALL PHASES
Medallions of Veal Sautéed with Sun-Dried Tomatoes, Shiitake Mushrooms, and Sweet Red Peppers	ALL PHASES
Romano-Crusted Lamb Chops Perfumed with Lemon and Rosemary	PHASE 2
Cold Smoked Filet Mignon with Field Mushrooms, Thyme, and Cabernet Wine Demi-Glace	PHASE 2

❧ Mallorca Restaurant ☞

1390 West 9th Street, Cleveland, OH 44113
(216) 687-9494, www.clevelandmallorca.com

As the name Mallorca suggests, this award–winning restaurant in Cleveland's Warehouse District offers the cuisine of Spain and Portugal. It provides a delicious option to the steakhouses and contemporary American cooking so readily found in this Midwestern city. The service at Mallorca is outstanding—the tuxedoed servers work efficiently and very professionally, but never hurry the diners. The portions are generous (so South Beach dieters need to be careful), and the entrées are served with fresh vegetables, rice, or Spanish potatoes. Your server will be happy to substitute more vegetables for the starches.

APPETIZERS, SOUPS, AND SALADS

Shrimp in Garlic Sauce	ALL PHASES
Mussels in Green Sauce	ALL PHASES
Mussels in Fra Diavolo Sauce	ALL PHASES
Clams in Marinara Sauce	ALL PHASES
Gazpacho	ALL PHASES
Garlic Soup	ALL PHASES
Spanish Vegetable Soup	PHASE 2

ENTRÉES

Shrimp in Garlic Sauce	ALL PHASES
Grilled Filet of Salmon	ALL PHASES
Filet of Sole with Clams, Mussels, and Shrimp in Green Sauce	ALL PHASES
Chicken Breast in a Garlic Sauce	ALL PHASES
Jumbo Shrimp in a White Wine Sauce	PHASE 2
Veal Scaloppine with Fresh Mushrooms in a Marsala Wine Sauce	PHASE 2
Veal Scaloppine with Roast Peppers in a Lemon-Wine Sauce	PHASE 2

❧ Sans Souci ❧

Renaissance Cleveland Hotel, Tower City Center
24 Public Square, Cleveland, OH 44113
(216) 696-5600, www.marriott.com

A premier dining destination in the heart of Cleveland, Sans Souci serves outstanding food that draws on Mediterranean cuisines, including those of France, Italy, Spain, Morocco, and Greece. Eclectic yet elegant, the award-winning menu changes often with the seasons and the markets, and there is an excellent wine list with interesting bottles from Spain and Italy. If you're looking for a quiet, relaxing restaurant, the sort of place that's good for talking business, this is it. The ground-floor setting in the historic Renaissance Cleveland Hotel overlooking Public Square features a huge stone fireplace, beamed ceilings, and hand-painted murals depicting country life in Provence.

APPETIZERS, SOUPS, AND SALADS

Sautéed Calamari with Baby Shiitakes	ALL PHASES
Beef Carpaccio	ALL PHASES
Wood-Grilled Mussels with Cilantro and Tomato Fondue	ALL PHASES
Gazpacho and Crab Salad	ALL PHASES
Seafood Minestrone	PHASE 3

ENTRÉES

Wood-Grilled Tuna with Roasted Eggplant	ALL PHASES
Oven-Roasted Cod with Clam Fumet	ALL PHASES
Whole-Wheat Penne Pasta with Broccoli Rabe, Asparagus, Tomatoes, and Ricotta "Pesto"	PHASE 2
Lamb Two Ways with Artichokes and Caramelized Root Vegetables	PHASE 3
Prosciutto-Wrapped Pork Tenderloin	PHASE 3

❦ XO Prime Steaks ❧

500 West St. Clair Avenue, Cleveland, OH 44113
(216) 861-1919, www.xoprimesteaks.com

XO Prime Steaks began life as a hip, trendy restaurant in Cleveland's Warehouse District. Today it's still hip and trendy, but it has been subtly transformed into an outstanding modern steakhouse. The steaks at XO are aged in the restaurant between 18 to 24 days, then seared in an imported broiler that can reach temperatures up to 2,500 degrees. If you order a steak, avoid the butter, blue cheese, and cream sauces, and select South Beach Diet–friendly Peppercorn Demi Roasted Garlic and Herb Sauce or the Red Wine Reduction to accompany it.

APPETIZERS AND SALADS

Jumbo Shrimp Cocktail	ALL PHASES
Beefsteak Tomato Salad	ALL PHASES
Traditional Caesar Salad (no croutons)	ALL PHASES
House Mixed Greens with Shaved Pears and Spicy Pecans	PHASE 2

ENTRÉES

Beef Filet (center cut, 8 oz)	ALL PHASES
Texas Sirloin (10 oz)	ALL PHASES
New York Strip (14 oz)	ALL PHASES
Free-Range Domestic Veal Chop	ALL PHASES
Thyme-Roasted Nova Scotia Salmon with Sautéed Arugula	ALL PHASES
Prosciutto-Wrapped Chilean Sea Bass	PHASE 3
Herb-Roasted Grouper with Sautéed Spinach and Preserved Lemon Butter	PHASE 3

SIDE DISHES

Sautéed Garlic Spinach	ALL PHASES
Caramelized Onions and Portobello Mushrooms	ALL PHASES
Sautéed Broccoli Rabe with Garlic and Chiles	ALL PHASES

❧ Abacus ❧

4511 McKinney Avenue, Dallas, TX 75205
(214) 559-3111, www.abacus-restaurant.com

Since it opened in 1999, Abacus has garnered award after award, and for good reason: This restaurant offers dishes that are a delicious, interesting, and eclectic blend of Mediterranean, Cajun/Creole, Southwestern, and Pacific Rim influences. The cooking here can best be described as contemporary global cuisine. It's all served in a sleek, casually elegant setting with three separate, art-filled dining rooms that are ideal for business entertaining. In addition to the Small and Big Plate offerings, there is sushi and sashimi (Phase 1 and 2 dieters should stick with the sashimi).

APPETIZERS

Kobe Beef Carpaccio with Baby Mâche	ALL PHASES
Seared Rare Ahi Tuna with Asparagus	ALL PHASES

ENTRÉES

Grilled Prime Lamb T-Bones with Rosemary Demi-Glace	PHASE 2
Wood-Roasted Buffalo Tenderloin on Red Wine Butter with Mixed Baby Veggies	PHASE 3
Pan-Seared Diver Sea Scallops with Gold Beets, Morel Mushrooms, and Lobster Sauce	PHASE 3
Pan-Seared Sea Bass with Lobster Mushrooms and Champagne Butter	PHASE 3

SIDE DISHES

Sautéed Forest Mushrooms	ALL PHASES
Grilled Asparagus	ALL PHASES
Steamed Edamame	ALL PHASES

❧ Dakota's Restaurant ❧

600 North Akard Street, Dallas, TX 75201
(214) 740-4001, www.dakotasrestaurant.com

To get into Dakota's Restaurant, diners have to take an elevator down to 18 feet below street level. The reason? The restaurant is on land once occupied by the First Dallas Baptist Church—and a clause in the deed forbade any future owner from serving alcohol on former church grounds. "On" isn't the same as "under," however, so the restaurant was placed below ground. The menu here is sophisticated steakhouse, with the emphasis on prime beef.

APPETIZERS AND SALADS

Shrimp Cocktail Stack with Cucumber Salad	ALL PHASES
Caesar Salad with Parmigiano-Reggiano (no croutons)	ALL PHASES
Red Oak Salad with Baby Shrimp	ALL PHASES
Diver Sea Scallops with Caramelized Pink Grapefruit, Lemon Beurre Blanc, and Celery Purée	PHASE 3

ENTRÉES

Scottish Salmon	ALL PHASES
Filet Mignon (8 oz)	ALL PHASES
New York Strip Steak (14 oz)	ALL PHASES
Australian Cold-Water Lobster Tails	ALL PHASES
Ahi Tuna with Orange Avocado Salad	PHASE 2

SIDE DISHES

Grilled Asparagus	ALL PHASES
Sautéed Broccoli Rabe	ALL PHASES
Butternut Squash Casserole	PHASE 3

❧ Javier's ❧

4912 Cole Avenue, Dallas, TX 75205
(214) 521-4211, www.javiers.net

There are no tamales or tacos on the menu here—the food at Javier's is what you might find at a fine restaurant in Mexico City, with service to match. This upscale yet casual restaurant has been serving authentic Mexican food in Dallas since 1977. The décor at Javier's has a true Mexican feeling, with tiled floors, dark wooden furniture, a spectacular copper-topped bar, and beautiful tapestries on the walls. For adventurous business travelers, Javier's is a good choice. The overall feel is intimate and welcoming, even though this popular Dallas institution is often crowded.

APPETIZERS, SOUPS, AND SALADS

Ceviche of White Fish and Shrimp	ALL PHASES
Guacamole	ALL PHASES
Spicy Chicken Consommé with Serrano Peppers, Onions, and Cilantro	ALL PHASES
Shrimp Salad with Sliced Avocados, Tomatoes, and Garbanzos	ALL PHASES
Black Bean Soup	ALL PHASES
Tortilla Soup	PHASE 3

ENTRÉES

Jumbo Shrimp in Special Diablo Sauce	ALL PHASES
Red Snapper in Garlic and Lemon Sauce	ALL PHASES
Mesquite-Smoked Chicken	ALL PHASES
Sautéed Tenderloin Filet in Black Pepper Sauce	ALL PHASES
Grilled Quail in Chile Ancho and Garlic Sauce	ALL PHASES
Sautéed Shrimp in Garlic and Lemon Sauce	ALL PHASES
Red Snapper Filet with Veracruz Sauce	ALL PHASES
Broiled Chicken with Mole Sauce	ALL PHASES
Grilled Chicken Breast with Butter and Lemon Juice	PHASE 3

❧ Sambuca Uptown ❧

2120 McKinney Avenue, Dallas, TX 75201
(214) 744-0820, www.sambucarestaurant.com

Live music seven nights a week and an eclectic menu distinguish this acclaimed restaurant, one of the first upscale places to open in uptown Dallas (there's also a Sambuca cousin in the Addison area). Sambuca features a stunning modern design with intimate dining areas, private rooms, and a delightful courtyard. The food covers a broad range of styles and ingredients, giving South Beach dieters a number of acceptable and very interesting choices.

APPETIZERS AND SALADS

Ceviche of Shrimp and Jumbo Lump Crab	ALL PHASES
Carpaccio of Beef Tenderloin and Yellowfin Tuna with Wasabi Sauce	ALL PHASES
House Salad of Tomato, Cucumber, Red Onion, and Feta	PHASE 2
Swiss Chard–Wrapped Beef with Mozzarella and Portobello Mushrooms	PHASE 3

ENTRÉES

Miso-Glazed Sea Bass with Bok Choy	ALL PHASES
Roast Rack of New Zealand Lamb with Fresh Vegetables	ALL PHASES
Filet of Beef Tenderloin on Wilted Greens (8 oz)	ALL PHASES
Peppercorn-Encrusted Yellowfin Tuna with Butternut Squash Ribs	PHASE 2
Crab-Stuffed Salmon with Roasted Root Vegetables	PHASE 3
Whisky-Injected Grilled Pork Chop with Ruby Red Port Wine Reduction	PHASE 3

SIDE DISHES

Steamed Asparagus with Lemon	ALL PHASES
Coriander and Fennel–Dusted Butternut Squash	PHASE 2

★ *Sambuca is also located in Atlanta.*

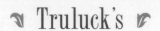

Truluck's

2401 McKinney, Dallas, TX 75201
(214) 220-2401, www.trulucks.com

Truluck's is so committed to fresh crab that the restaurant operates its own fisheries off Naples, Florida. Stone crab is a specialty here, and the rest of the menu shows the same concern for fresh ingredients carefully prepared. The cuisine at Truluck's draws from cooking styles covering the globe. The menu is extensive and very interesting, with a wide variety of dishes South Beach dieters can happily enjoy.

APPETIZERS, SOUPS, AND SALADS

Oysters on the Half Shell	ALL PHASES
Shrimp Cocktail	ALL PHASES
Seared Ahi Tuna	ALL PHASES
Chilled Alaskan King Crab with Mustard Sauce	ALL PHASES
North Atlantic Jonah Stone Crab Claws	ALL PHASES
Sonoma Greens Salad with Maytag Blue Cheese	ALL PHASES
Spicy Crab and Artichoke Soup	PHASE 2

ENTRÉES

Jonah Stone Crab Platter with Steamed Broccoli	ALL PHASES
Center-Cut Tenderloin Filet (8 oz)	ALL PHASES
Pan-Seared Alaskan Halibut with Sautéed Garlic Spinach	ALL PHASES
Pan-Seared Diver Scallops with Sautéed Green Beans	ALL PHASES
Seared Sesame-Crusted Tuna with Tamari Wine Sauce	PHASE 2

SIDE DISHES

Steamed Broccoli	ALL PHASES
Steamed Asparagus	ALL PHASES
Steak Mushrooms	ALL PHASES

❧ The American Restaurant ❧

Crown Center Complex
25th Street and Grand Avenue, Kansas City, MO 64108
(816) 545-8000, www.americanrestaurantkc.com

The American Restaurant was designed in 1974 as a world-class show-case to anchor the new Crown Center Complex. It's been succeeding in its mission ever since, providing fine American food in a spectacular setting. Guests enter the dining room from a dramatic staircase; once seated, they can enjoy panoramic views of downtown Kansas City through the massive windows. The award-winning cooking (menus change daily) at The American Restaurant matches the views—this is one of the finest restaurants in the Midwest and a great place to take business associates.

APPETIZERS AND SALADS

Flash-Broiled Scallops	ALL PHASES
Mixed Baby Greens with Buttermilk-Sage Dressing (no croutons)	ALL PHASES
Red Oak Lettuces with Manchego Cheese and Cinnamon Almonds	PHASE 2

ENTRÉES

Sautéed Loup de Mer	ALL PHASES
Ginger-Crusted Escolar with Miso Soup	ALL PHASES
Roasted Lamb Loin with Eggplant Caviar	PHASE 2
Pan-Roasted Halibut with Grilled Organic Vegetables and Sweet Corn Sauce	PHASE 2
Four-Hour Veal Shank	PHASE 2
Grilled Black Angus Filet with Trumpet Mushrooms and Autumn Squash	PHASE 2

SIDE DISHES

Sautéed Sonoma Mushrooms	ALL PHASES

❧ Pierpont's at Union Station ☙

30 West Pershing Road, Kansas City, MO 64108
(816) 221-5111, www.herefordhouse.com

The jewel of the renovated Union Station, Pierpont's has the décor of 1914—dark mahogany, ornamental plaster, and lots of marble—but the cuisine of contemporary times. The casual but elegant atmosphere is complemented by outstanding service and a wine list offering an unusually good selection of half bottles and glasses. Although beef has pride of place on the menu here, as befits a Kansas City restaurant, Pierpont's offers some other interesting dishes that will appeal to South Beach dieters. Skip the mashed potatoes and potato pancakes that come with certain entrées.

APPETIZERS AND SALADS

Shrimp Cocktail	ALL PHASES
"Knife & Fork" Caesar Salad (no croutons)	ALL PHASES
Spinach Salad with Serrano Ham and Fresh Goat Cheese	PHASE 2
Crispy Root Vegetable Salad	PHASE 3

ENTRÉES

Petite Tenderloin with Artichoke Hearts and Asparagus	ALL PHASES
Tenderloin Filet (7 oz)	ALL PHASES
Rotisserie Half Chicken with Tarragon Jus and Sautéed Zucchini	ALL PHASES
Kurobuta Pork Loin with Red Wine Onion Syrup	PHASE 2

SIDE DISHES

Asparagus	ALL PHASES
Artichoke Hearts	ALL PHASES
Baby Green Beans	ALL PHASES
Mushrooms	ALL PHASES
Julienne Zucchini	ALL PHASES

❧ Plaza III ☙

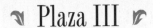

4749 Pennsylvania Avenue, Kansas City, MO 64112
(816) 753-0000, www.plazaiiisteakhouse.com

Consistently recognized as one of the Top 10 steakhouses in America, Plaza III is a Kansas City institution dating back to 1963. This restaurant serves up not only a signature Kansas City strip steak (South Beach dieters need to be careful of the huge portion here), but also signature Kansas City jazz, live every evening Wednesday through Saturday. The expansive wine list offers more than 700 bottles. Plaza III features excellent service to go along with the outstanding cooking, making this a top choice for business dining.

APPETIZERS AND SALADS

Jumbo Shrimp Cocktail	ALL PHASES
Hand-Chopped Tenderloin Tartare with Golden Caviar	ALL PHASES
Caesar Salad (no croutons)	ALL PHASES

ENTRÉES

Filet Mignon (8 oz)	ALL PHASES
Prime Kansas City Strip Steak (14 oz)	ALL PHASES
Double-Cut Lamb Rib Chops	ALL PHASES
Double Breast of Chicken with Lemon and Herbs	ALL PHASES
Fresh Atlantic Salmon	ALL PHASES

SIDE DISHES

Sautéed Fresh Spinach	ALL PHASES
Steamed Fresh Asparagus	ALL PHASES
Grilled Seasonal Vegetables with Herb Butter	PHASE 3
Sautéed Fresh Whole Mushrooms in Seasoned Butter Sauce	PHASE 3

❧ Ruth's Chris Steak House ☙

The Plaza Steppes
700 West 47th Street, Suite 115, Kansas City, MO 64112
(816) 531-4800, www.ruthschris.com

Back in 1965, a struggling young single mother named Ruth Fertel mortgaged her house to buy a place called Chris Steak House in New Orleans. She knew nothing about the restaurant business, but what she lacked in experience she made up for in intelligence, hard work, and natural instinct. Ruth's Chris Steak House, as the restaurant came to be known, soon became one of the most popular destinations in town, a gathering place for great food, quality service, and a warm atmosphere. Today Ruth's Chris Steak Houses are found in 88 locations worldwide, including 30 in the United States. The Kansas City branch is an outstanding representative of the chain in a city made famous by beef. Ask for the vegetable side dishes to be steamed and served without sauces.

APPETIZERS, SOUPS, AND SALADS

Shrimp Cocktail	ALL PHASES
Sliced Tomato and Onion with Blue Cheese Crumbles	PHASE 2
Louisiana Seafood Gumbo	PHASE 3

ENTRÉES

Petite Filet (8 oz)	ALL PHASES
Petite Filet Topped with Jumbo Gulf Shrimp	ALL PHASES
Veal Chop with Sweet and Hot Peppers	ALL PHASES
Ahi Tuna Stack Topped with Colossal Lump Crabmeat	ALL PHASES

SIDE DISHES

Fresh Asparagus	ALL PHASES
Fresh Steamed Broccoli	ALL PHASES
Fresh Spinach	ALL PHASES

★ *Ruth's Chris Steak House is also located in Atlanta, Boston, Chicago, Cleveland, Dallas, Las Vegas, Minneapolis, New York City, Orlando, San Francisco, and Washington, DC.*

❧ Starker's Reserve ☙

201 West 47th Street, Kansas City, MO 64112
(816) 753-3565, www.starkersreserve.com

Upscale yet comfortable and traditional, Starker's Reserve Restaurant offers contemporary American cuisine in an uncrowded, intimate atmosphere. This is a very attractive restaurant, with excellent service and a menu that changes daily according to the seasons and the markets. The wine cellar has been winning awards regularly since 1992—the by-the-glass selection is particularly strong. Attention to detail in both the kitchen and the dining room pays off well here, making Starker's Reserve one of the better choices for a quiet evening.

SOUPS AND SALADS

Chanterelle Mushroom Soup	ALL PHASES
Hearts of Romaine Caesar Topped with Pecorino Shavings and Anchovies (no croutons)	ALL PHASES
Leaf Lettuce Salad with Granny Smith Apples, Maytag Cheese, and Pommery Mustard Vinaigrette	PHASE 2

ENTRÉES

Grilled Rack of Lamb with Zucchini and Great Northern Beans in Sweet Basil Pesto Broth	ALL PHASES
Seasonal Vegetable Offering	ALL PHASES
Pan-Roasted Veal Chop with Sweet Corn and Fava Bean Succotash	PHASE 3
Grilled Alaskan Salmon with Ten Chile Pico De Gallo and Sweet Corn Cream	PHASE 3

SIDE DISHES

Grilled Asparagus	ALL PHASES
Sautéed Chanterelle Mushrooms	ALL PHASES
Garlic Sautéed Spinach	ALL PHASES
Corn and Fava Bean Succotash	PHASE 3

❧ Bradley Ogden ☞
at Caesars Palace

3570 Las Vegas Boulevard South, Las Vegas, NV 89109
(702) 731-7410, www.caesars.com

Bradley Ogden grew to cooking fame with his top-ranked California restaurants, including his signature restaurant, The Rock Creek Inn, in Marin County. Personable and outgoing, Ogden is a popular guest on cooking shows. This restaurant, his first venture outside of California, features his outstanding "farm fresh" American cuisine. In fact, in 2004 it was the first restaurant in Las Vegas to ever receive the prestigious "Best New Restaurant" award from the James Beard Foundation. The menu here varies considerably, depending on what's available at local markets. The daily specials are always interesting and often feature regional specialties.

APPETIZERS, SOUPS, AND SALADS

Bradley's Caesar Salad (no croutons)	ALL PHASES
Market Salad	PHASE 2
Autumn Vegetable Soup	PHASE 2
Duet of Asparagus	PHASE 2

ENTRÉES

Steamed Alaskan Halibut with Ingrid's Maine Lobster and Asparagus	ALL PHASES
Triple-Seared "Kobe Style" New York Strip (8 oz)	ALL PHASES
Wood-Fired Kurobuta Pork Loin	ALL PHASES
Wisconsin Pheasant with Cauliflower, Grapes, and Chanterelles	PHASE 2
Lightly Roasted Sturgeon with Diced Beets	PHASE 3

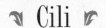 Cili

At Bali Hai Golf Club
5160 Las Vegas Boulevard South, Las Vegas, NV 89119
(702) 856-1000, www.cili.com

Enter Cili and enter a Balinese paradise with South Pacific décor, designed to be in keeping with the Bali Hai Golf Club. The cuisine here is basically regional American with strong influences from Thailand and the Pacific Rim. There are dishes that will appeal to South Beach dieters in all phases, but be sure to read the menu descriptions carefully and avoid items that are high in saturated fat from butter and cheese.

APPETIZERS AND SALADS

Beef Carpaccio with Roasted Pepper Aïoli	ALL PHASES
Balinese-Style Chicken and Beef Satays	ALL PHASES
Tuna Tataki with Chinese Mustard Sauce	ALL PHASES
Smoked Chicken Soup with Broccoli and Black Beans	ALL PHASES
Wild Mushroom Soup	ALL PHASES
Field Greens Salad with White Balsamic Vinaigrette	ALL PHASES

ENTRÉES

Chicken Diablo with Fire-Roasted Onions, Bell Peppers, and Sautéed Rapini	ALL PHASES
Alaskan Halibut with Green Beans and Shallots	ALL PHASES
Seared Veal T-Bone with Grilled Asparagus and Whole-Grain Mustard Sauce	ALL PHASES
Tandoori Lamb Chops with Eggplant Salad	ALL PHASES
Grilled Pork Chops with Broccoli au Gratin	PHASE 3
Seared Atlantic Salmon with Parsnip Purée	PHASE 3

SIDE DISHES

Sautéed Spinach	ALL PHASES
Sautéed Asparagus	ALL PHASES
Sautéed Green Beans	ALL PHASES

❧ The Eiffel Tower Restaurant ☞

Paris Hotel
3655 Las Vegas Boulevard South, Las Vegas, NV 89109
(702) 948-6937, www.eiffeltowerrestaurant.com

The Eiffel Tower Restaurant is located, naturally enough, on the 11th floor of the replica of the famed tower found at the Paris Hotel. Guests are whisked to the restaurant in a glass elevator that opens into the bustling activity of the kitchen. They are then escorted to the stunning dining room, where panoramic views of the city immediately grab the attention. The menu features modern updates of classic French dishes, making this a fine destination for South Beach dieters.

APPETIZERS

Cold Smoked Salmon with Condiments	ALL PHASES
Black Pepper–Marinated Raw Beef with Mustard Aïoli	ALL PHASES
Sautéed Casco Bay Sea Scallops	ALL PHASES
Cracked Corn, Wild Mushrooms, and Escargot Provençale	PHASE 3

ENTRÉES

Sautéed Wild Red Snapper, Broccoletti, and Confit Onion	ALL PHASES
Braised Turbot, Vegetables, and Bouillabaisse Broth	ALL PHASES
Filet of Wild Sea Bass with Herb Coulis and Roasted Cauliflower	ALL PHASES
Roasted and Braised Farm-Raised Organic Chicken	ALL PHASES
Roasted Rack of Lamb with Tarragon Jus	ALL PHASES
Sautéed Veal Medallions with Wild Forest Mushrooms	ALL PHASES
Filet of Atlantic Salmon with Pinot Noir Sauce	PHASE 2
Sautéed Venison Medallions with Huckleberry Sauce	PHASE 3

SIDE DISHES

Sautéed Wild Mushrooms	ALL PHASES
Sautéed Spinach	ALL PHASES
Asparagus with Brown Butter	PHASE 3

❧ Tsunami Asian Grill ❧

The Venetian Resort Hotel Casino
3355 Las Vegas Boulevard South, Las Vegas, NV 89109
(702) 414-1980, www.venetian.com

Tsunami Asian Grill may overlook the replica Grand Canal (complete with gondolas and singing gondoliers) and St. Mark's Square area at the Venetian Hotel complex, but the décor and food here have nothing to do with Italy. The interior of Tsunami is sleek and modern, with a massive bar and imaginative Asian imagery on the walls. The innovative Pacific Rim menu draws from the culinary traditions of Thailand, Japan, Korea, and other Asian cuisines. South Beach dieters dining here for business should stay away from the extensive selection of sake and choose wine instead.

APPETIZERS, SOUPS, AND SALADS

Steamed Edamame Finished with Organic Sea Salt	ALL PHASES
Miso Soup with Wakame Seaweed and Soft Tofu	ALL PHASES
Warm Vegetable and Tofu Salad, Boiled Egg, and Curry Peanut Sauce	PHASE 2
Mandarin Orange Chicken Salad with Sesame Ginger	PHASE 2
Garlic Chicken Lettuce Wrap with Water Chestnut, Mushrooms, and Ponzu Soy Sauce	PHASE 2
Chili Lime Beef Salad, Cucumber, and Papaya Dressed with Orange Yuzu	PHASE 2

ENTRÉES

Fiery Mongolian Beef with Scallions, Sweet Onions, and Roasted Arbol Chili	ALL PHASES
Togarashi-Crusted Hawaiian Mahi Mahi with Mango Salsa	PHASE 2
Sambal Goreng Shrimp with Bell Peppers and Opal Basil in Green Coconut Curry	PHASE 3

❧ Valentino ❧

The Venetian Resort Hotel Casino
3355 Las Vegas Boulevard South, Las Vegas, NV 89109
(702) 414-3000, www.venetian.com

Racks holding some 24,000 bottles of fine wine from around the world line the walls at Valentino. Not surprisingly, the wine cellar here has won a number of awards. So has the cuisine. The food is contemporary Italian—innovative, yet true to its Old World roots. In classic Italian style, the dishes are made using only the finest and freshest of ingredients, which are often flown in from Italy if necessary. South Beach dieters have plenty of options at Valentino.

APPETIZERS AND SALADS

Star Anise–Flavored Atlantic Salmon with Fennel Brulée	PHASE 2
Alaskan King Crab with Parsnip, Salsify, Tomato, and Arugula	PHASE 2

ENTRÉES

Broiled Mediterranean Branzino Served over Mashed Garbanzo Beans with Herb-Flavored Vincotto Reduction	ALL PHASES
Shellfish Medley Baked in Broth with Mixed Vegetables	ALL PHASES
Grilled "Kurobuta" Pork Chops with Smoked Braised Cabbage and Pork Demi-Glace	ALL PHASES
Colorado Lamb T-Bone Steaks with Rhubarb Sauce and Sautéed Sunchokes	PHASE 2
Ahi Tuna Crusted in Almonds with an Orange-Flavored Foam	PHASE 2
Pan-Roasted Veal Delmonico with Black Pepper Crust, Vin Santo and Marion Berry Sauce, and Fennel Gratin	PHASE 3

❧ Campanile ❧

624 South La Brea Avenue, Los Angeles, CA 90036
(323) 938-1447, www.campanilerestaurant.com

This elegant restaurant takes its name from the Mediterranean-style villa, complete with bell tower (campanile) and courtyard, that is its home. The French- and Italian-influenced cuisine at Campanile emphasizes fresh, locally grown ingredients. The menu is broad, with a wide range of fish and shellfish choices, as well as elegant versions of classic dishes, such as grilled prime rib.

APPETIZERS AND SALADS

Chef's Creek and Hama Hama Oysters	ALL PHASES
Bibb Lettuce and Herb Salad with Lemon Vinaigrette	ALL PHASES
Wild Mushroom Frisée Salad	ALL PHASES
Octopus and Squid Salad	ALL PHASES

ENTRÉES

Sautéed Baby Sole with Soy Beans	ALL PHASES
Seared Rare Big-Eye Tuna with Crushed Shelling Beans	ALL PHASES
Grilled Wild Alaskan Halibut with Mussels, Clams, Shrimp, and Saffron Aïoli	ALL PHASES
Wild Alaskan King Salmon with Baby Artichokes and Preserved Lemon	ALL PHASES
Grilled Prime Rib with Bitter Greens and Shelling Bean Ragout	ALL PHASES
Roasted Kurobuta Pork Chop with Sautéed Hedgehog Mushrooms and Roasted Peaches	PHASE 2

SIDE DISHES

Sautéed Beet Greens	ALL PHASES
Roasted Tricolor Cauliflower	ALL PHASES

❧ Nick and Stef's Steakhouse ❧

330 South Hope Street, Los Angeles, CA 90071
(213) 680-0330, www.patinagroup.com

Voted best steakhouse in downtown Los Angeles, Nick and Stef's is the creation of restaurateur Joachim Splicha (the restaurant name comes from his twin sons). Though the dining room is modern, what you'll find at Nick and Stef's is a traditional steakhouse, featuring delicious dry-aged beef. The menu also offers some excellent nonbeef choices, including a number of fish, chicken, and vegetable dishes. South Beach Diet beef-lovers should choose the lower-fat steak cuts, such as the petit filet mignon.

APPETIZERS AND SALADS

Grilled Jumbo Shrimp Cocktail	ALL PHASES
Signature Tableside-Prepared Caesar Salad (no croutons)	ALL PHASES
Bluefin Tuna and Prime Filet with Yuzu, Soy, and Mirin	PHASE 2
Baby Arugula Leaves with Shaved Market Pear, Spiced Walnuts, and Pecorino Cheese	PHASE 2

ENTRÉES

Oakwood-Grilled King Salmon Steak with Haricot Verts and Stewed Shallots	ALL PHASES
American Kobe-Style Beef Hanger Steak (8 oz)	ALL PHASES
Herb-Crusted Boneless Rib Medallion (8 oz)	ALL PHASES
Petit Filet Mignon (6 oz)	ALL PHASES
All-Natural Pork Chop (12 oz)	ALL PHASES
Grilled Farm-Raised Chicken Split in Half	ALL PHASES
Roasted Free-Range Chicken Breast with Grapes, Chanterelles, and Spinach	PHASE 2

SIDE DISHES

Sautéed Forest Mushrooms	ALL PHASES
Sautéed Baby Bok Choy with Soy and Chili	ALL PHASES
Marinated Heirloom Tomatoes with Shaved Onion	ALL PHASES

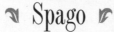 Spago

176 North Canon Drive, Beverly Hills, CA 90210
(310) 385-0880, www.wolfgangpuck.com

The flagship of chef Wolfgang Puck's restaurant empire, Spago in Beverly Hills is one of LA's finest restaurants. The menu emphasizes imaginative international fare based on French, Asian, and Californian influences. The seasonal dishes are made using the freshest local ingredients whenever possible. While some menu offerings come with potatoes or rice, the kitchen is happy to accommodate South Beach dieters with extra vegetables instead. Diners can watch the activity in the kitchen through a huge wall of colorful etched glass. This restaurant is extremely popular—so make reservations in advance.

APPETIZERS, SOUPS, AND SALADS

Broiled Japanese Black Cod with Hijiki Seaweed Salad	ALL PHASES
Marinated Japanese Hamachi and Tuna Sashimi	ALL PHASES
Austrian Chicken Bouillon with Julienne Vegetables	ALL PHASES
Vegetable Minestrone	PHASE 3
Fresh Burata Mozzarella Salad with Ice Wine Vinaigrette	PHASE 3

ENTRÉES

Pan-Roasted French Turbot with Ragout of Vegetables	ALL PHASES
Wild Striped Bass with Littleneck Clams and Sautéed Spinach	ALL PHASES
Seared Rare "Big Eye" Tuna with Crushed Shelling Beans	ALL PHASES
Pan-Roasted Organic Chicken with Oregon Morel Mushrooms	ALL PHASES
Steamed Wild Alaskan Salmon "Hong Kong Style"	ALL PHASES
Grilled Bone-In Prime Kansas City Steak with Sautéed Baby Turnips and Radishes	PHASE 2

★ *Spago is also located in Las Vegas.*

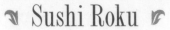 Sushi Roku

8445 West 3rd Street, West Hollywood, CA 90048
(323) 655-6767, www.sushiroku.com

In addition to an unusually broad range of sushi and sashimi offerings, Sushi Roku offers dinner entrées that combine traditional Japanese cooking with a California touch. The beautiful dining room reflects modern Japanese style and features authentic Asian woods and hand-made bamboo tables. The outdoor dining patio has a cascading water-fall and tranquil pond. The emphasis on very fresh fish at this elegant restaurant makes it an excellent choice for anyone on the South Beach Diet. Skip the white rice, and enjoy the organic garden salad instead.

APPETIZERS AND SALADS

Sautéed Sesame Gobo (Burdock Root)	ALL PHASES
Renkon (Lotus Root)	ALL PHASES
Oshinko (Pickled Japanese Vegetables)	ALL PHASES
Organic Garden Salad with Japanese Dressing	ALL PHASES
Hijiki Salad	ALL PHASES

ENTRÉES

Alaskan King Salmon Sashimi with Japanese Vinaigrette	ALL PHASES
Baked Oysters with Oriental Miso Sauce	ALL PHASES
Maine Lobster Ceviche with Organic Teardrop Tomatoes	ALL PHASES
Pan-Roasted Lobster, Shrimp, and Scallop with Garlic Peppercorn	ALL PHASES
Sautéed Baby Abalone in Garlic Soy	ALL PHASES
Japanese Conch Escargot Bourguignon Style	PHASE 2
Chilean Sea Bass with Mixed Mushrooms in Citrus Sauce	PHASE 2
Tamari-Glazed Quail with Snow Peas and Banashemeji Mushrooms	PHASE 2
Salmon Sashimi and Jalapeño Tempura with Garlic Ponzu Sauce	PHASE 3

★ *Sushi Roku is also located in Las Vegas.*

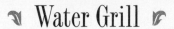 Water Grill

544 South Grand, Los Angeles, CA 90071
(213) 891-0900, www.watergrill.com

Fresh fish and shellfish are givens in a city with a long coastline, but Water Grill, conveniently located in downtown Los Angeles, carries the term *fresh* even further. The seafood at this restaurant is of the highest possible quality; to preserve flavor, it's prepared simply using the finest ingredients. Not surprisingly, the menu changes daily. The dining room is in an elegant Art Deco style with soft lighting and an intimate table arrangement that's ideal for business dining.

APPETIZERS AND SALADS

Oysters on the Half Shell	ALL PHASES
Maine Lobster	ALL PHASES
Oregon Dungeness Crab	ALL PHASES
Mexican White Shrimp	ALL PHASES
Tuna Tartare with Crushed Avocado, Pink Radish, and Green Peppercorn Vinaigrette	ALL PHASES
Hamachi Sashimi	ALL PHASES
Peekytoe Crab Salad with Satsuma Tangerine, Ruby Grapefruit, and Mimosa Gelée	PHASE 2

ENTRÉES

Slow-Steamed Alaskan Halibut with Spiced Artichokes and Kalamata Olive Purée	ALL PHASES
Wild John Dory with Pearl Onions and Sweet Basil	ALL PHASES
Poached Salmon with Sunchoke Purée, Fava Beans, English Peas, and Black Trumpet Mushroom Vinaigrette	PHASE 2

❧ Acqua ☙

Four Seasons Hotel Miami
1435 Brickell Avenue, Miami, FL 33131
(305) 358-3535, www.fourseasons.com

Serving fine Italian food in an elegant setting, Acqua is located off the seventh-floor main lobby of the luxurious Four Seasons Hotel in downtown Miami. The food here has an authentic Mediterranean feel that's very appropriate for the South Florida setting. There are plenty of delicious options among the entrées—just ask your server to substitute more vegetables for the potatoes that accompany many dishes. Acqua is a sophisticated restaurant with outstanding, highly professional service and an excellent wine list.

APPETIZERS AND SALADS

Beef Carpaccio with Shaved Parmigiano-Reggiano, Lemon, and Olive Oil	ALL PHASES
Seared Jumbo Scallops with Spumante Sauce	PHASE 2
Grilled Vegetable and Goat Cheese Timbale with Baby Romaine Salad and Pine Nuts	PHASE 2
Bocconcini of Mozzarella with Marinated Tomato Salad and Caprese Dressing	PHASE 3

ENTRÉES

Seared Branzino with Sautéed Spinach, Cherry Tomato, and Black Olives	ALL PHASES
Roasted Free-Range Chicken Breast with Lavender and Lemon Glaze	ALL PHASES
Roasted Yellow Snapper with Blue Crab and Prosecco Sauce	PHASE 2
Grilled Beef Tenderloin with Barolo Sauce	PHASE 2
Entrecôte Florentine, Grilled with Herbs, Garlic Butter, and Portobello Mushrooms	PHASE 3

❧ Blue Door ☙
Restaurant & Brasserie

Delano Hotel
1685 Collins Avenue, Miami Beach, FL 33139
(305) 674-6400, www.delano-hotel.com

The Delano Hotel in Miami Beach is the creation of famed hotelier Ian Schrager. This is the place to go for celebrity-spotting and people-watching in a beautiful, all-white setting. For this restaurant, chef Claude Troisgros designed an appropriate menu that combines innovative interpretations of traditional American fare with tropical accents from Brazil and elsewhere. South Beach dieters will have to be careful of the complex sauces that are a feature of many of the dishes. The Brasserie, with its comfortable, living room–style furniture, is more relaxed and casual, while the Blue Door Terrace is ideal for al fresco dining day or night.

APPETIZERS AND SALADS

Seared Rare Yellowfin Tuna with Marinated Daikon	ALL PHASES
Avocado Guacamole and Blue Crab Salad	ALL PHASES

ENTRÉES

Pan-Seared Red Snapper in Saffron and Dill Sauce	ALL PHASES
Colorado Lamb Loin and Oven-Roasted Eggplant with Tomato Confit	ALL PHASES
Grilled Beef Tenderloin in a Garlic and Rosemary Crust with Yuca Galette and Cabernet Bordelaise Sauce	PHASE 2
Filet of Black Grouper in Brown Butter Sauce with Caramelized Baby Fennel	PHASE 3
Marinated Loin of Venison with Peppercorn Red Wine Sauce, Chestnuts, and Celery Purée	PHASE 3

❧ Joe's Stone Crab ☙

11 Washington Avenue, Miami Beach, FL 33139
(305) 673-0365, www.joesstonecrab.com

No visit to Miami is complete without a meal at Joe's Stone Crab. This landmark restaurant, founded in 1913, was the first—and for a long time the only—restaurant in South Beach. Times have changed in South Beach, however: Joe's is still in its original place but has expanded, and a bustling scene has grown up around it. The specialty of the house since the 1920s has been stone crab claws with Joe's special mustard sauce, and so it remains, although other seafood, steaks, and chicken are available for those who wish. Joe's is open only from mid-October through the end of July; stone crabs are only available until mid–May. No reservations are taken, and diners are seated on a first-come, first-serve basis. It's worth the wait.

APPETIZERS

Shrimp Cocktail	ALL PHASES
Oysters on the Half Shell	ALL PHASES
Prince Edward Island Mussels in a Spicy Tomato Broth	ALL PHASES

ENTRÉES

Stone Crabs with Joe's Mustard Sauce	ALL PHASES
Cold Seafood Platter	ALL PHASES
Grouper with Sun-Dried Tomato, Artichoke, and Almonds	ALL PHASES
Seafood Cioppino with Mussels, Shrimp, Lobster, Grouper, Clams, and Stone Crabs in Spicy Tomato Broth	ALL PHASES
Prime Top Sirloin (8 oz)	ALL PHASES
Half Spring Chicken	ALL PHASES

SIDE DISHES

Broccoli	ALL PHASES
Sautéed Mushrooms	ALL PHASES
Sautéed Spinach	ALL PHASES

★ *Joe's Stone Crab is also located in Chicago and Las Vegas.*

❧ Pacific Time ❧

915 Lincoln Road, Miami Beach, FL 33139
(305) 534-5979, www.pacifictimerestaurant.com

The Asian Pacific food at Pacific Time is fused with the cuisines of Indonesia, Vietnam, and India. In the wrong hands, this could result in clashing flavors and novelty for its own sake, but at Pacific Time, chef/owner Jonathan Eismann combines the ingredients in imaginative ways that meld them into exciting new tastes. The menu is based on local produce and seafood, and it changes daily—at any time nearly half the dishes are based on what's available at the market that day. Located in a large loftlike space, with a high ceiling and mahogany furnishings, the restaurant is a stylish addition to the Lincoln Road area of South Beach. It's a great place for dinner after enjoying the unique retailers and art galleries nearby.

APPETIZERS AND SALADS

Yellowfin Tuna Tataki	ALL PHASES
Citrus-Cured Salmon Tartare	ALL PHASES
Market Salad with Miso Ginger Vinaigrette	ALL PHASES
Pacific Time Miso Rubbed Chicken Salad	ALL PHASES
Indochine Beef Salad with Chinese Cabbage	ALL PHASES
Hijiki and Hyashi Wakame Seaweed Salad	ALL PHASES

ENTRÉES

Aromatic Steamed Pacific Halibut	ALL PHASES
Pan-Broiled Dry-Aged Colorado Beef	ALL PHASES
Herb-and-Truffle-Roasted Farm Chicken with Natural Shiitake Jus	ALL PHASES
Grilled Colorado Lamb Chops with Field Greens	ALL PHASES
Szechuan-Grilled Local Mahi-Mahi	PHASE 2

❧ Prime 112 ☙

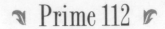

The Browns Hotel
112 Ocean Drive, Miami Beach, FL 33139
(305) 532-8112, www.prime112.com

One of the trendiest restaurants in all of South Beach, Prime 112 is an outstanding steakhouse located in the newly restored, historic The Browns Hotel. Dating back to 1915, The Browns was the first hotel on Miami Beach. Prime 112 is an interesting contrast to the historic setting, with its sleek, contemporary, but comfortable design, modern menu, and relaxing background music. Steak is the focal point of the menu here—stay away from the butter toppings and go for the Prime 112 steak sauce, the chimichurri sauce, or the cabernet sauce instead. For those who don't eat meat, there's also a good selection of imaginatively prepared fresh seafood. Because Prime 112 is so popular, reservations are needed well in advance.

APPETIZERS AND SALADS

Maine Lobster Cocktail	ALL PHASES
Beefsteak Tomato and Onion Salad	ALL PHASES
Organic Field Greens with Shaved Pear	PHASE 2

ENTRÉES

Filet Mignon (8 oz)	ALL PHASES
New York Strip Steak (14 oz)	ALL PHASES
Seared Center Cut Yellowfin Tuna with Avocado, Hearts of Palm, and Kumamoto Oyster Sauce	ALL PHASES
Grilled Local Grouper with Melted Leeks, Fresh Tomato and Basil Aïoli	ALL PHASES
Soy-Marinated Sea Bass with Steamed Baby Bok Choy	ALL PHASES

SIDE DISHES

Grilled Asparagus	ALL PHASES
Sautéed Spinach	ALL PHASES
Sautéed Broccoli Rabe	ALL PHASES
Sautéed Forest Mushrooms	ALL PHASES

❧ Cosmos Restaurant ❧

Graves 601 Hotel
601 First Avenue North, Minneapolis, MN 55403
(612) 677-1100, www.cosmosrestaurant.com

In 2005 executive chef Seth Daugherty of Cosmos was named Best New Chef in the Nation by *Food & Wine* magazine. The menu at this sleek restaurant is why—it's a highly creative approach to contemporary American cuisine. The fresh ingredients, drawn from local suppliers whenever possible, are carefully prepared and impeccably served. This restaurant is an outstanding choice for a South Beach Diet–friendly business dinner—or a special occasion meal.

APPETIZERS AND SALADS

Carpaccio of Lamb	ALL PHASES
Ahi Tuna Tartare with Cilantro Sesame Vinaigrette	ALL PHASES
Cosmos Lettuce Blend with Roast Shallots	ALL PHASES
Sesame Poached Sea Scallop with Asian Pear and Wakame Seaweed	PHASE 2
Lobster Tail with Avocado, Mango, and Arugula	PHASE 2
Heirloom Tomato with Buffalo Mozzarella	PHASE 3

ENTRÉES

Pan-Seared Five-Spice Grouper with Miso Citrus Broth	ALL PHASES
Pan-Roasted Breast of Chicken with White Beans, Chanterelle Mushrooms, and English Peas	PHASE 2
Grilled Lamb Chop with Watercress, Preserved Lemon, Currant, and Goat Cheese	PHASE 2
Pan-Seared Duck Breast	PHASE 3

❧ Manny's Steakhouse ☙

Hyatt Regency
1300 Nicollet Mall, Minneapolis, MN 55403
(612) 339-9900, www.mannyssteakhouse.com

Consistently voted one of the top steakhouses in the nation, Manny's has great food and a classic steakhouse feel: dark wood, leather, and a bustling ambience. This is no place for vegetarians, but those who would prefer not to eat steak at Manny's can find a reasonable choice of other entrées. Main courses at Manny's come unaccompanied—skip the potatoes and choose salad or a vegetable as your side dish.

APPETIZERS AND SALADS

Oysters on the Half Shell	ALL PHASES
Shrimp Cocktail	ALL PHASES
Caesar Salad	ALL PHASES
Hearts of Palm	ALL PHASES
Sliced Tomato and Onion	ALL PHASES
Mixed Greens	ALL PHASES
Sliced Tomato and Mozzarella	PHASE 3

ENTRÉES

Filet Mignon (10 oz)	ALL PHASES
Lamb Chops	ALL PHASES
Veal Loin Chop	ALL PHASES
Lemon Pepper Chicken	ALL PHASES

SIDE DISHES

Sautéed Mushrooms	ALL PHASES
Asparagus	ALL PHASES
Broccoli	ALL PHASES

❧ Mission American ☙ Kitchen & Bar

IDS Center
77 South Seventh Street, Minneapolis, MN 55402
(612) 339-1000, www.missionamerican.com

This spacious, comfortable restaurant offers a simple and beautifully prepared menu and supplements it with an excellent wine list. This is the sort of restaurant that pleases everyone—it's a good place for a date, a family celebration, or a business meal. The selection of side vegetables is excellent here, so South Beach dieters shouldn't hesitate to ask the server to substitute vegetables for the potatoes that accompany most dishes.

APPETIZERS, SOUPS, AND SALADS

Deviled Eggs	ALL PHASES
Baja Ceviche (no chips)	ALL PHASES
Seared Tuna with Orange, Fennel, and Chili Lemon Zest	PHASE 2
Roasted Grape and Goat Cheese Salad	PHASE 2
Chili-Coated Goat Cheese with Figs	PHASE 3

ENTRÉES

Halibut Steak	ALL PHASES
Grilled Pork Tenderloin with Greens and Garlic Sauce	ALL PHASES
Grilled Lamb Chops with Ratatouille	ALL PHASES
Grilled Pork Chop	ALL PHASES
Roasted Chicken with Arugula Bread Salad	PHASE 3

SIDE DISHES

Grilled Asparagus	ALL PHASES
Broccoli Sautéed with Garlic	ALL PHASES
Grilled Portobello Mushrooms	ALL PHASES
Spicy Green Beans	ALL PHASES

❧ The Oceanaire Seafood Room ☙

Hyatt Regency
1300 Nicollet Mall, Minneapolis, MN 55403
(612) 333-2277, www.theoceanaire.com

Journey back to the swank feel of a 1930s ocean liner in this retro supper club. The illusion is thorough, down to the white-jacketed servers and red leather booths. The food at The Oceanaire is fresh seafood, flown in from around the world. The menu varies daily, depending on what's available on the international market. Whatever dish you choose, it's prepared simply to bring out the pure flavors.

APPETIZERS

House-Cured Salmon	ALL PHASES
Jumbo Shrimp Cocktail	ALL PHASES
Steamed Mussels à la Marinière	ALL PHASES
Grilled Calamari	ALL PHASES
Fresh Crabmeat Cocktail	ALL PHASES

ENTRÉES

Dayboat Alaskan Halibut "T-Bone"	ALL PHASES
Columbia River Chinook Salmon "Captain's Cut"	ALL PHASES
Gulf of Mexico Red Snapper	ALL PHASES
"Fin and Shell" Fish Stew with Spicy Tomato Fumé	ALL PHASES
Grilled Cape Neddick Sea Scallops with American Lobster Sauce	ALL PHASES
Broiled Shrimp Scampi	ALL PHASES

SIDE DISHES

Green Beans Amandine	ALL PHASES
Sautéed Spinach and Mushrooms	ALL PHASES

★ *The Oceanaire Seafood Room is also located in Atlanta, Dallas, and Washington, DC.*

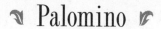 Palomino

LaSalle Plaza
825 Hennepin Avenue, Minneapolis, MN 55402
(612) 339-3800, www.palomino.com

Conveniently close to the Hennepin theater district, Palomino offers European-inspired regional American cuisine. The ambience here is stylish, but the prices are reasonable. This is a good place for dining with business clients, a pretheater dinner, or an after-theater snack. The menu offers an unusually wide selection of acceptable dishes for South Beach dieters. Just be sure to skip the tempting butter sauces.

APPETIZERS AND SALADS

Brick Oven–Roasted Mussels	ALL PHASES
Brick Oven–Roasted Clams	ALL PHASES
Grilled Tiger Prawns with Sun-Dried Tomatoes and Fresh Basil	ALL PHASES
Greek Salad (no croutons)	ALL PHASES
Caesar Salad (no croutons)	ALL PHASES
Baby Field Greens with Chèvre and Pumpkin Seeds	PHASE 2

ENTRÉES

Grilled Seafood Louie (includes grilled salmon, bay shrimp, and Dungeness crab)	ALL PHASES
Greek Salad with Rotisserie Chicken	ALL PHASES
Spit-Roasted Chicken	ALL PHASES
Spit-Roasted Pork Loin with Fennel Rosemary Crust	ALL PHASES
Grilled Wild Mushroom Salad with Toasted Walnuts and Crumbled Gorgonzola	PHASE 2
Asiago-Almond-Crusted Sea Scallops	PHASE 2
Pan-Roasted Chicken Marsala	PHASE 2
Pan-Seared Chicken with Wild Mushroom Stuffing	PHASE 3

★ *Palomino is also located in Dallas, Los Angeles, and San Francisco.*

❧ DB Bistro Moderne ☙

55 West 44th Street, New York, NY 10036
(212) 391-2400, www.danielnyc.com

The initials DB stand for famed chef Daniel Boulud. In this restaurant, Boulud reinterprets the traditional French bistro and brings it into the 21st century, merging French cuisine with the fresh flavors of American markets. The menu reflects the changing seasons and focuses on the simplicity of fine ingredients. The end result is exactly what the restaurant's name promises: creative cooking presented in a modern, comfortable environment.

APPETIZERS AND SALADS

Moroccan Tuna Tartare with Cucumber Raita, Chickpeas, and Harissa	ALL PHASES
Maine Lobster Salad with Mesclun, Heart of Palm, Green Beans, and Pesto Dressing	ALL PHASES
Peekytoe Crab Salad with Grapefruit Gelée, Citrus Segments, and Avocado	PHASE 2
Tomato Tarte Tatin with Goat Cheese Frisée and Black Olives	PHASE 3

ENTRÉES

Grilled Yellowfin Tuna with "One Minute Vegetables," Shiitake Mushrooms, and Lemon Grass Vinaigrette	ALL PHASES
Organic Chicken Breast with Chanterelles and Chicken Jus	ALL PHASES
Roasted Maine Halibut with Artichoke-Fava Bean Fricassee, Tomato Confit, and Provençale Vegetables	PHASE 2

SIDE DISHES

Vegetables Jardinière	ALL PHASES
Super Green Spinach	ALL PHASES

❧ Fresco by Scotto ☙

34 East 52nd Street, New York, NY 10022
(212) 935-3434, www.frescobyscotto.com

The Scotto family, including local news anchor Rosanna Scotto, owns and runs this relaxed, friendly, northern Italian restaurant. The slogan here is "Italian comfort food," and the Scotto family means it—portions are large and the welcome is warm, making it a favorite lunch spot for executives based in midtown Manhattan. The clan appears often on NBC's *Today* show, demonstrating their Tuscan cuisine. If you're on Phase 3, start your meal the Italian way with a half order of one of their homemade pastas.

APPETIZERS

Vegetable Antipasto	ALL PHASES
Manila Clams with Roasted Tomatoes, Barlotti Beans, and Arugula	ALL PHASES
Homemade Mozzarella and Marinated Roasted Peppers	PHASE 3

ENTRÉES

Roasted Capon Breast with Sun-Dried Tomato and Fresh Herbs	ALL PHASES
Grilled Veal Chop with Cremini Mushrooms	ALL PHASES
Spiced, Seared, and Sliced Yellowfin Tuna with Roasted Baby Artichokes and Wild Mushrooms	ALL PHASES
Pan-Roasted Branzino Filet with Roasted Butternut Squash, Spinach, and Wild Mushrooms	PHASE 2

SIDE DISHES

Sautéed Broccoli Rabe with Roasted Garlic, Oregano, and Cherry Tomatoes	ALL PHASES
Stewed String Beans all' Amatriciana	ALL PHASES
Pan-Roasted Wild Mushrooms with Shallots	ALL PHASES

❧ Gramercy Tavern ❧

42 East 20th Street, New York, NY 10003
(212) 477-0777, www.gramercytavern.com

This popular dining establishment serves outstanding American cuisine. The more casual Tavern Room at the front doesn't take reservations and serves a simpler menu, which you can eat at the bar, if you like. The three main antique-filled dining rooms are more formal and quieter. At lunch, dishes in the dining rooms can be ordered à la carte; at dinner, three different prix fixe menus prevail. Because Gramercy Tavern is a particularly good spot for a business lunch, the dishes listed below are from the dining room lunch menu. Check the Web site for dinner options, which change often.

APPETIZERS AND SALADS

Tuna Tartare with Cucumber, Arugula, Sesame, Coriander, and Sea Urchin Vinaigrette	ALL PHASES
Chilled Lobster with Hearts of Palm, Avocado, Shiso, and Yuzo Vinaigrette	ALL PHASES

ENTRÉES

Striped Bass with Minced Autumn Vegetables, Wild Spinach, and Ginger	ALL PHASES
Roasted Cod with Brandade, Braised Squash, Olive Tapenade, and Tomato Vinaigrette	ALL PHASES
Organic Chicken with Roasted Greenmarket Vegetables	ALL PHASES
Braised Shoulder of Lamb with Tomato Tart and Autumn Waxed Beans	PHASE 3
Salt-Baked King Salmon with Braised Lobster Mushrooms, Bok Choy, and Corn	PHASE 3

Molyvos

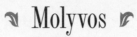

Wellington Hotel
871 7th Avenue, New York, NY 10019
(212) 582-7500, www.molyvos.com

The closest you can get to Greece in New York is Molyvos, a large and lively taverna only one block south of Carnegie Hall. The dishes here are traditional Greek cuisine updated for contemporary American diners, and the authenticity comes through in every dish. The many appetizers on the menu represent traditional Greek mezedes, or small plates. Entrées are typically served with potatoes or rice, which South Beach diners can replace with vegetables. The service is attentive but unobtrusive, making Molyvos a good choice for a quiet meal.

APPETIZERS AND SALADS

Fruit-Wood-Grilled Baby Octopus	ALL PHASES
Citrus-Marinated Scallops	PHASE 2
Greek Garden Salad with Olives and Feta Cheese	PHASE 2
Sampling of Traditional Greek Spreads (eggplant salad, "caviar" mousse, and cucumber yogurt with garlic)	PHASE 2
Mediterranean Vegetable Stew with Gigantes Beans	PHASE 2

ENTRÉES

Grilled Fish with Roasted Vegetables	ALL PHASES
Lemon and Garlic Roast Chicken with Spinach and Tomato	ALL PHASES
Grilled Baby Lamb Chops with Wood-Grilled Eggplant Salad	ALL PHASES
Braised Savory Marinated Lamb Shanks with Orzo, Tomatoes, and Kefalotryi Cheese	PHASE 3

SIDE DISHES

Sautéed Spinach	ALL PHASES
Braised Wild Greens	ALL PHASES

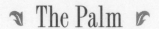 The Palm

837 2nd Avenue, New York, NY 10017
(212) 687-2953, www.thepalm.com

The Palm on Second Avenue is the flagship location of this famed steakhouse restaurant group. The walls of this venerable restaurant—it dates back to 1926 and has always been at this address—are covered with caricatures of local notables and national celebrities. The food and atmosphere at The Palm haven't changed much over time, perhaps because the grandsons of the founders still run the restaurant. This is a place for great steaks and a relaxed good time.

APPETIZERS AND SALADS

Hearts of Palm	ALL PHASES
Caesar Salad	ALL PHASES
Chopped Tomato and Onion Salad	ALL PHASES
Clams on the Half Shell	ALL PHASES
Oysters on the Half Shell	ALL PHASES
Jumbo Shrimp Cocktail	ALL PHASES

ENTRÉES

Prime Aged New York Strip (12 oz)	ALL PHASES
Filet Mignon (10 oz)	ALL PHASES
Lamb Chops	ALL PHASES
Salmon Fillet	ALL PHASES
Tuna Steak	ALL PHASES
Swordfish Steak	ALL PHASES

SIDE DISHES

String Beans	ALL PHASES
Broccoli	ALL PHASES
Leaf Spinach	ALL PHASES

★ *The Palm is also located in Atlanta, Boston, Chicago, Dallas, Las Vegas, Los Angeles, Miami, Orlando, and Washington, DC.*

◄ Christini's Ristorante Italiano ►

7600 Dr. Phillips Boulevard, Orlando, FL 32819
(407) 345-8770, www.christinis.com

Owner Chris Christini has been offering outstanding cooking and his personal charm at Christini's Ristorante Italiano for more than 40 years—and for all that time, this has consistently been one of Orlando's finest restaurants. The traditional Tuscan cuisine is outstanding, and there's an unusually good choice of wines by the glass. The Old World feeling is enhanced by highly professional service in a lovely dining room complete with strolling musicians. For a business dinner, Christini's may be one of the best choices in town.

APPETIZERS AND SALADS

Portobello Mushrooms Sautéed with Balsamic Vinegar	ALL PHASES
Carpaccio of Filet Mignon	ALL PHASES
Marinated Anchovies with Sweet Fresh-Roasted Peppers and Onions	ALL PHASES
Arugula Salad with Celery Root, Fennel, and Gorgonzola Cheese	PHASE 2
Sautéed Jumbo Gulf Shrimp with Pernod and Barolo	PHASE 2

ENTRÉES

Broiled Filet of Norwegian Salmon on Baby Greens	ALL PHASES
Assorted Seafood in a Vegetable-Flavored Fish Broth	ALL PHASES
Broiled Australian Lobster Tail with Garlic and Lemon	ALL PHASES
Rack of Lamb with Balsamic Mint Sauce	ALL PHASES
Grilled Veal Paillard	ALL PHASES
Veal Scaloppine Sautéed with Fresh Mushrooms, Shallots, and Marsala	PHASE 2
Boneless Breast of Chicken Sautéed with Peas, Artichokes, Shiitakes, and White Wine	PHASE 2

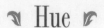 Hue

629 East Central Boulevard, Orlando, FL 32801
(407) 849-1800, www.huerestaurant.com

The management at Hue describes the cuisine as progressive American, which seems to mean traditional American with a pan-Asian twist. However it's described, the food here is excellent, served in a candlelit setting with high ceilings, large windows, and exposed columns. There is also a large outdoor patio for more casual dining. The menu changes daily to reflect what's freshest in the market. Nearly all the entrées come with chive mashed potatoes and a mélange of sautéed vegetables; ask your server for extra vegetables, and skip the potatoes if you're on Phase 1 or 2.

APPETIZERS AND SALADS

U-12 Shrimp Cocktail, with a Trio of Sauces	ALL PHASES
Pan-Asian Chop Chop: Tamari Chicken, Romaine, Pickled Ginger, Red Peppers, and Macadamia Nuts in a Sesame Ginger Vinaigrette	ALL PHASES
Roasted Scallops with Chili Garlic Mayo	ALL PHASES
Beef Tataki and Cucumber Salad	ALL PHASES

ENTRÉES

Wood-Grilled All-Natural Chicken	ALL PHASES
Oven-Roasted Chilean Sea Bass with Asiago Tapenade	PHASE 2
Wood-Grilled Lamb Rack with Mint Demi-Glace	PHASE 2
Center Cut Filet Mignon with Red Wine Demi-Glace	PHASE 2
Wood-Grilled Salmon with Sesame Hoisin Glaze	PHASE 3

❧ Jack's Place ❧

The Rosen Plaza Hotel
9700 International Drive, Orlando, FL 32819
(407) 996-9700, www.rosenplaza.com

Only minutes away from major Orlando attractions such as SeaWorld and Universal Orlando and adjacent to the Orange County Convention Center, Jack's Place at the Rosen Plaza Hotel offers a varied menu featuring prime steaks and fresh seafood. The atmosphere is casual yet elegant, with gracious service, and the décor is fascinating—the walls are lined with hundreds of caricatures of famous people who once strolled through the lobby of New York's Waldorf-Astoria Hotel. The drawings were done by Jack Rosen, father of owner Harris Rosen, who named the hotel in his father's honor.

APPETIZERS AND SALADS

Shrimp Cocktail with Lemon and a Duet of Sauces	ALL PHASES
Grilled Crab Cake with Red Pepper Black Bean Relish	ALL PHASES
Caesar Salad (no croutons)	ALL PHASES
Mixed Field Greens with Wild Strawberries and Fresh Mozzarella	PHASE 3

ENTRÉES

Jack's Little Italy Steak with Arugula and Balsamic Glaze	ALL PHASES
Blackened Filet Mignon (8 oz) with Roasted Garlic Sauce	ALL PHASES
Roasted Rack of Lamb with Dijon Mustard Persillade	ALL PHASES
Rock Cornish Game Hen with Sun-Dried Cherry Sauce	PHASE 2
Chicken Sautéed with Marinated Tomatoes and Fresh Mozzarella	PHASE 3
Seared Halibut Meunière with Fennel, Dill, and Pine Nuts	PHASE 3

SIDE DISHES

Sautéed Forest Mushrooms	ALL PHASES
Julienne Vegetables with Herbs of Provence	ALL PHASES

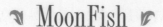 MoonFish

7525 West Sand Lake Road, Orlando, FL 32819
(407) 363-7262, www.fishfusion.com

Fish fusion is the theme at MoonFish, where the innovative cuisine is based on fresh seafood from around the world. For those who aren't in the mood for fish, the restaurant also offers prime steaks cooked over a natural citrus and oak wood–fired pit (the steaks are big enough to share). The food is complemented by a wine list of more than 300 labels, also drawn from around the world. The menu at MoonFish varies daily, depending on what seafood is freshest at the markets. The preparation methods also change to best suit each type of fish or shell-fish, so ask your server for details before ordering.

APPETIZERS

Wood-Roasted Oysters	ALL PHASES
Seared Rare Tuna Sashimi	ALL PHASES
MoonFish Seafood Cocktail	ALL PHASES

ENTRÉES

Bamboo Steamer with Lobster Tail, King Crab, Fish, Shrimp, and Steamed Fresh Vegetables	ALL PHASES
Bouillabaisse with Lobster, King Crab, Shrimp, and Fish	ALL PHASES
Shrimp and Scallop Scampi with Lobster Vegetable Consommé	ALL PHASES
Miso-Glazed Chilean Sea Bass	ALL PHASES
Filet Mignon (12–13 oz)	ALL PHASES

SIDE DISHES

Oak-Grilled Asparagus	ALL PHASES
Szechuan Green Beans	ALL PHASES
Wok-Steamed Ginger Veggies	ALL PHASES

❧ Todd English's bluezoo ☛

Walt Disney World Swan & Dolphin Hotel
1500 Epcot Resort Boulevard, Lake Buena Vista, FL 32830
(407) 934-1111, www.thebluezoo.com

Charismatic chef and cookbook author Todd English is the moving force behind this very enjoyable restaurant, located within a whimsical hotel at the Walt Disney World Resort. The amazing dining room, decorated with iridescent bubbles of hand-blown glass and a school of aluminum fish swimming behind the bar, sets the stage for an award-winning menu. Needless to say, seafood is the specialty here—diners can watch it being grilled to perfection in the exhibition kitchen on the circular "dancing fish" rotisserie.

APPETIZERS AND SALADS

Garlic-Roasted Jumbo Shrimp	ALL PHASES
Selection of Maine Lobster Tail, Oysters, Clams, Jumbo Shrimp, and Tuna Tartare	ALL PHASES
Yellowfin Tuna Tartare	ALL PHASES
Salad of Greens with Apple and Avocado	PHASE 2
Vietnamese Crab Salad with Melon and Mango	PHASE 3

ENTRÉES

Simply Fish (daily selection grilled on teppanyaki grill)	ALL PHASES
This Evening's Dancing Fish	ALL PHASES
Seared Nori Wrapped Tuna with Gingered Greens	ALL PHASES
Flame-Grilled Tenderloin of Beef Filet	ALL PHASES
Miso-Glazed Chilean Sea Bass with Pea Tendril Salad	ALL PHASES

SIDE DISHES

Zaatar Spice Roast Carrots	PHASE 2

❧ Eleven Eleven Mississippi ☙

1111 Mississippi, St. Louis, MO 63104
(314) 241-9999, www.1111-m.com

Located in the heart of the beautiful Lafayette Square neighborhood in a restored historic warehouse, this casual but elegant restaurant features dishes baked in an oak-fired brick oven. The cuisine here is influenced by Tuscany and northern California, so the end result is a restaurant with the feel of a rustic wine country bistro just minutes from downtown St. Louis. The open kitchen, gleaming hardwoods, brick, copper, and two open fireplaces create a warm and cozy atmosphere that nicely complements the excellent wine cellar and innovative cooking. South Beach dieters should ask for extra vegetables instead of the potatoes or pasta that come with some dishes.

APPETIZERS, SOUPS, AND SALADS

Grilled Portobello with Spinach and Roasted Pepper Vinaigrette	ALL PHASES
Chilled Heirloom Tomato Gazpacho	ALL PHASES
Mixed Field Greens with Red Onion, Pine Nuts, Tomatoes, and Pecorino Cheese	PHASE 2

ENTRÉES

Grilled Chicken Breast with Smoked Tomato Vinaigrette and Sautéed Spinach	ALL PHASES
Seared Mahi Mahi with Wilted Swiss Chard	ALL PHASES
Grilled Salmon with Caper Tomato Relish	ALL PHASES
Frittata with Peppers, Onions, Tomatoes, and Crumbled Goat Cheese	PHASE 2
Pork Tenderloin with Black Mission Fig Demi-Glace	PHASE 3

SIDE DISHES

Grilled Asparagus with Melted Provolone and Sherry Vinaigrette	PHASE 2

❧ Lucas Park Grille and Market ☞

1234 Washington Avenue, St. Louis, MO 63103
(314) 241-7770, www.lucasparkgrille.com

This hot new restaurant bills itself as a steakhouse. That's a bit mis-
leading for two reasons. First, the restaurant also offers plenty of fresh
seafood—not surprising, because the chef grew up working on fishing
boats. Second, the cuisine here goes beyond standard steakhouse—
eclectic American would be a good way to describe it. The 8,000-
square-foot space was once a turn-of-the-century industrial building;
the spectacular double-high ceilings and oversized windows remain.
The careful renovation includes working stone fireplaces, comfy
couches, a huge bar, and a gourmet market, along with lovely views of
Lucas Park.

APPETIZERS AND SALADS

Beef Tenderloin Carpaccio	ALL PHASES
Vanilla-Scented Shrimp Ceviche Cocktail with Papaya and Avocado	PHASE 2
House Salad of Mixed Greens, Shaved Fennel, Roma Tomatoes, and Goat Cheese	PHASE 2
Caprese Salad of House-Made Mozzarella and Farm Tomatoes	PHASE 3

ENTRÉES

Grilled Marinated Steak with Smoked Wild Mushrooms	ALL PHASES
Beef Tenderloin Filet (8 oz)	ALL PHASES
Cast-Iron-Roasted Salmon with Wilted Spinach and Wild Mushrooms	ALL PHASES
Pan-Seared Halibut with Sea Beans and Spinach Salad	ALL PHASES
Cast-Iron-Roasted Free-Range Chicken with Spicy Pan Gravy	PHASE 3

❧ Mike Shannon's ☙
Steaks and Seafood

100 North 7th Street, St. Louis, MO 63101
(314) 421-1540, www.shannonsteak.com

The quality of the aged beef and the succulent seafood at this classic steakhouse keep guests coming back often. Co-owned by a former Cardinals third baseman, the restaurant features more than 500 photos of sports greats. True baseball fans come Friday and Saturday evenings after Cardinals home games to be there for Mike Shannon's live broadcast of his sports radio talk show. This relaxed steakhouse has a nice, family atmosphere, and there's always the chance of spotting a visiting sports celebrity.

APPETIZERS AND SALADS

Mussels Mediterranean	ALL PHASES
Shrimp Cocktail	ALL PHASES
Mixed Field Greens Salad	ALL PHASES
Salad of Tomato, Red Onion, and Fresh Couturier Cheese	PHASE 2

ENTRÉES

Strip Sirloin (12 oz)	ALL PHASES
Tenderloin Filet (8 oz)	ALL PHASES
Mint Garlic Broiled Chicken Breast	ALL PHASES
Steamed Oriental Salmon	ALL PHASES
Twin Lobster Tails	ALL PHASES

SIDE DISHES

Fresh Asparagus	ALL PHASES
Green Beans Amandine	ALL PHASES
Steamed Broccoli	ALL PHASES

◥ Mosaic ◤

1101 Lucas Avenue, St. Louis, MO 63101
(314) 621-6001, www.mosaictapas.com

Much of the menu at this stunning restaurant (with a focus on Pacific Rim fusion cuisine) is tapas style, so bring friends and try a variety of small dishes—in moderation if you're a South Beach dieter. The cuisine here combines classical European technique with the variety and freshness of ingredients available in American markets. The result is a restaurant with a wide-ranging menu. The visual experience at Mosaic is part of the fun. The building is a former factory; the modern design incorporates the original high ceilings and tall windows and adds a free-standing serpentine bar. The restaurant takes its name from the beautiful mosaic wall that dominates the dining room—an appropriate metaphor for the intriguing fusion cuisine.

APPETIZERS AND SALADS

Carpaccio of Beef with Toasted Hazelnuts	ALL PHASES
Tuna Tartare	ALL PHASES
Tuscan Broccoli Salad with Toasted Pine Nuts and Mustard Vinaigrette	ALL PHASES
Sake-Cured Atlantic Salmon	PHASE 2
Lobster Salad with Guacamole and Valencia Oranges	PHASE 2

ENTRÉES

Grilled Beef Kebab with Garlic Spinach and Harissa	ALL PHASES
Breast of Free-Range Chicken with Basil Pesto	ALL PHASES
Roasted Sea Scallop with Braised Leeks, Shaved Beef, and Chimichurri Sauce	ALL PHASES
Freshwater Prawns with Seaweed Salad and Tomato Ragout	ALL PHASES
Seared Tuna with Fava Beans, Wild Ramps, and Lemon Garlic Aïoli	PHASE 2

❧ SqWires ☙

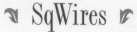

1415 South 18th Street, St. Louis, MO 63104
(314) 865-3522, www.sqwires.com

Named for the old Western Wire Factory it's housed in on historic
Lafayette Square, this popular restaurant features novel interpretations
of classic American cuisine. The seasonal menu offers fresh seafood and
prime meats, all imaginatively and carefully prepared (ask for vegetables to accompany the grilled meats). The unusual setting preserves
many of the fascinating 19th-century details of the building, including
the overhead factory pulley system and industrial fans.

APPETIZERS AND SALADS

Oysters on the Half Shell	ALL PHASES
Sesame Tuna Carpaccio with Wasabi Cilantro Aïoli	ALL PHASES
Roasted Garden Vegetable Salad	ALL PHASES
Shrimp and Avocado Salad	ALL PHASES
Ratatouille	ALL PHASES
Seafood Salad	ALL PHASES

ENTRÉES

Shrimp and Veggie Stir-Fry	ALL PHASES
Curry-Seared Scallops with Field Greens and Fresh Asparagus	ALL PHASES
Pepita-Seared Wild Salmon Topped with Black Bean Avocado Relish	ALL PHASES
Seafood Bouillabaisse	ALL PHASES
Grilled Strip Steak	ALL PHASES
Grilled Pork Tenderloin	ALL PHASES

❧ Aqua ☙

252 California Street, San Francisco, CA 94111
(415) 956-9662, www.aqua-sf.com

Upscale, sophisticated, innovative, and beautiful, Aqua is one of the finest dining experiences in San Francisco. The cuisine here is contemporary French, based on the abundance of seafood and local produce found in the San Francisco Bay area. The service and food presentation at Aqua are unbeatable, and the restaurant also offers an excellent wine list. The menu here changes often to reflect the current season and the best foods available. A South Beach dieter will have no trouble finding plenty to enjoy at this fine restaurant.

APPETIZERS, SOUPS, AND SALADS

Tartare of Ahi Tuna with Moroccan Spices	ALL PHASES
Hearts of Baby Romaine with Shaved Vegetables and Banyuls Vinegar	ALL PHASES
King Salmon Carpaccio with Beets	PHASE 3
Coachella Valley Corn Soup with Maine Scallop and Smoked Oyster	PHASE 3

ENTRÉES

Yellowfin Tuna with Rock Shrimp, Calamari, and Clams	ALL PHASES
Hawaiian Walu with Charmoula, Yogurt, and Grilled Leeks	ALL PHASES
Monkfish "Persillade" with Organic Peach, Cipollini Onion, Porcini, and Purslane	PHASE 2
Scottish Salmon with Pommery Mustard, Green Apples, and Endive	PHASE 2
White Sturgeon en Papillote with Speck Ham and Swiss Chard	PHASE 3

❧ Bob's Steak & Chop House ☙

Omni San Francisco Hotel
500 California Street, San Francisco, CA 94104
(415) 273-3085, www.bobs-steakandchop.com

Bob's Steak & Chop House is a little piece of Texas in California. This top-rated steakhouse has a clubby atmosphere, with rich mahogany booths and attentive service. The central location in the elegant Omni Hotel near Union Square makes this a good choice for business dining, whether it's dinner or a power breakfast. The traditional steakhouse menu prevails at Bob's—and it's done perfectly. Ask to substitute vegetables for the glazed carrots and potatoes that accompany the entrées. And skip the butter sauces on the broiled fish.

APPETIZERS AND SALADS

Shrimp Cocktail	ALL PHASES
Asparagus Salad with Roasted Peppers on a Bed of Mixed Greens	ALL PHASES
Beefsteak Tomato and Red Onion Salad with Crumbled Aged Blue Cheese	ALL PHASES

ENTRÉES

Prime Filet Mignon (9 oz)	ALL PHASES
New York Strip Steak (12 oz)	ALL PHASES
Pork Chops	ALL PHASES
Veal Chop (14 oz, bone in)	ALL PHASES
Broiled Salmon	ALL PHASES
Broiled Shrimp Scampi	ALL PHASES

SIDE DISHES

Fresh Broccoli	ALL PHASES
Sautéed Spinach and Mushrooms	ALL PHASES
Fresh Asparagus	ALL PHASES

★ *Bob's Steak & Chop House is also located in Dallas.*

❧ Boulevard ☙

One Mission Street, San Francisco, CA 94105
(415) 543-6084, www.boulevardrestaurant.com

Located in the historic 1889 French-style Audiffred Building, Boulevard's décor is classic Belle Epoque. The restaurant's hearty and flavorful American regional cuisine is moderated by traditional French influences. It emphasizes fresh, locally produced ingredients and an attractive presentation. In addition to the outstanding food (every entrée comes with a wide range of remarkable accompaniments too complex to describe here), the excellent waitstaff and extensive wine list make this a favorite of business diners.

APPETIZERS AND SALADS

Green Goddess Dungeness Crab Salad	ALL PHASES
Ahi Tuna and Hamachi Carpaccio	ALL PHASES
Seared Day Boat Sea Scallops with Point Reyes Clams	ALL PHASES
Star Route Organic Greens with White Nectarines, Gorgonzola, and Pine Nuts	PHASE 2

ENTRÉES

Pan-Seared Northern Halibut	ALL PHASES
Pan-Roasted Fresh Maine Cod Fish	ALL PHASES
Grilled Wild Pacific White Sea Bass	ALL PHASES
Wood Oven–Roasted Berkshire Pork Loin Chop	ALL PHASES
Wood Oven–Roasted Lamb Loin	ALL PHASES
Fire-Roasted Angus Filet Mignon	ALL PHASES

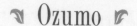 Ozumo

161 Steuart Street, San Francisco, CA 94105
(415) 882-1333, www.ozumo.com

The serenely beautiful dining room at Ozumo features stylish modern furniture, handmade lampshades, and wallpaper—and stunning views of San Francisco Bay. It's all a backdrop for the outstanding Japanese cuisine, including some intriguing dishes that incorporate French influences. In addition to a range of cold and hot appetizers and salads, and the offerings from the sushi bar (South Beach dieters need to stick to sashimi on Phases 1 and 2), Ozumo has a charcoal robata grill menu that features a variety of unusual small plates.

APPETIZERS AND SALADS

Kani Kani Kani: Chef's-Style Tofu and Dungeness Crab Cake with Spinach Aïoli	ALL PHASES
Futago: Thinly Sliced Beef Tenderloin with Garlic Sautéed Spinach and Japanese Eggplant	ALL PHASES
Aoba Salad: Watercress, Endive, Baby Romaine, Mizuna, and Cucumbers with Miso-Caesar Dressing	ALL PHASES
Hanabi: Slices of Hamachi and Avocado with Warm Ginger and Jalapeño Ponzu Sauce	PHASE 2

ENTRÉES

Maguro: Big-Eye Tuna with Hijiki Seaweed	ALL PHASES
Yasai Vegetables: Grilled Bamboo Shoots, White Asparagus, Japanese Eggplant, Zucchini, and Snap Peas	ALL PHASES
Jidori: Charcoal-Broiled Chicken Skewers with Spicy Miso and Yuzu Pepper	ALL PHASES
Hitsuji: Lamb Chops with Herb Pesto	ALL PHASES
Burikama: Yellowtail Collar with Spicy Seaweed Garlic Ponzu Sauce	PHASE 2
Gyu Fillet: Charcoal-Broiled Beef Fillet with Shiitake Mushrooms and Madeira Sauce	PHASE 2

❧ Restaurant Gary Danko ❧

800 North Point Street, San Francisco, CA 94109
(415) 749-2060, www.garydanko.com

Cosmopolitan and elegant, Restaurant Gary Danko is one of the most highly rated restaurants in San Francisco. The California cuisine here is sophisticated and contemporary, created with the finest locally produced ingredients and centered on lively dishes that change with the seasons. Dinners here are on a prix fixe basis, with a choice of three, four, or five courses. Artisanal cheeses from around the world are a specialty—sampling them is acceptable for South Beach dieters on Phase 2 or Phase 3.

APPETIZERS AND SALADS

Glazed Oysters with Osetra Caviar	ALL PHASES
Seared Ahi Tuna with Avocado, Nori, Enoki Mushrooms, and Lemon Soy Dressing	ALL PHASES
Heirloom Tomato Salad with Lemon-Caper Dressing and Black Olive-Pine Nut Gremolata	ALL PHASES
Corn and Arugula Salad with Parmigiano-Reggiano and Tomato Vinaigrette	PHASE 3

ENTRÉES

Pan-Seared Sea Scallops with Piquillo Peppers and Onion Confit	ALL PHASES
Horseradish-Crusted Salmon Medallion with Dilled Cucumbers	ALL PHASES
Moroccan Spiced Squab with Chermoula	ALL PHASES
Herb-Crusted Loin of Lamb with Israeli Couscous and Yellow Zucchini	PHASE 2
Pan-Seared Branzini with Red Pepper Succotash and Wilted Arugula	PHASE 2

❧ 1789 Restaurant ☞

1226 36th Street, NW, Washington, DC 20007
(202) 965-1789, www.1789restaurant.com

One of the top tables in America according to *Gourmet* magazine, 1789 Restaurant is located in a renovated Federal townhouse in Washington's historic Georgetown district. The relaxed country inn ambience in the five dining rooms is accented by American antiques, period prints, and Limoges china. The menu here is equally elegant, with generous portions of traditional and new American dishes presented beautifully by attentive waiters. It's a perfect venue for entertaining business clients or for celebrating a special occasion.

APPETIZERS AND SALADS

Prince Edward Island Mussels in Fennel Garlic Broth	ALL PHASES
Field Greens with Mustard Tarragon Vinaigrette	ALL PHASES
Classic Caesar Salad (no croutons)	ALL PHASES
Nantucket Bay Scallop Margarita with Tequila Ice	PHASE 2
Grilled Quail on a Wilted Salad of Radicchio, Taleggio Cheese, Prosciutto, and Fennel	PHASE 3

ENTRÉES

Rack of American Lamb with Garlic Spinach and Rosemary Shiraz Sauce	PHASE 2
Sake-Marinated Yellowfin Tuna with Wild Mushroom Ginger Broth	PHASE 2
Veal Loin with Bitter Orange Glaze, Asparagus, and Oven-Dried Tomatoes	PHASE 2
Chesapeake Rockfish on Roasted Red Pepper Sauce with Porcini Mushroom Flan	PHASE 3
Pine Nut–Crusted Chicken with Portobello Mushrooms, Roasted Peppers, Prosciutto, and Goat Cheese	PHASE 3

❦ The Capital Grille ❧

601 Pennsylvania Avenue, NW, Washington, DC 20004
(202) 737-6200, www.thecapitalgrille.com

The Capital Grille in Washington, DC, is part of a high-end chain with locations in a number of major cities. Visiting this one, in the nation's capital, is particularly appropriate. The atmosphere here is relaxed elegance and style. The Capital Grille serves perfectly prepared classic steakhouse offerings, emphasizing prime beef aged on the premises (hold the butter and cheese sauces). The service is excellent, the dining room is clubby and private, and the menu is complemented by a good wine list with over 300 selections.

APPETIZERS AND SALADS

Cold Shellfish Platter	ALL PHASES
Shrimp Cocktail	ALL PHASES
Smoked Norwegian Salmon with Dill Mayonnaise	ALL PHASES
The Grille's Steak Tartare	ALL PHASES
Prosciutto-Wrapped Mozzarella with Vine-Ripe Tomatoes	PHASE 3

ENTRÉES

Kona-Crusted Dry-Aged Sirloin	ALL PHASES
Sliced Filet Mignon with Cipollini Onions and Sautéed Wild Mushrooms	ALL PHASES
The Grille's Signature Veal Chop	ALL PHASES
Split Roasted Chicken with Spicy Red Rub Spices	ALL PHASES
Fresh Grilled Swordfish with Asparagus, Spinach, Corn, and Smoky Roasted Tomatoes	PHASE 3

SIDE DISHES

Roasted Seasonal Mushrooms	ALL PHASES
The Grille's Fresh Vegetables	ALL PHASES

★ *The Capital Grille is also located in Atlanta, Boston, Chicago, Dallas, Kansas City, Las Vegas, Miami, Minneapolis, and New York City.*

❧ Ceiba ❧

701 14th Street, NW, Washington, DC 20005
(202) 393-3983, www.ceibarestaurant.com

The name *Ceiba* (pronounced SAY-bah) pays tribute to the imposing, umbrella-shaped tree found throughout the New World tropics. Given the name, it's no surprise to find that this restaurant serves contemporary Latin American cuisine. Indeed, the cooking of the Yucatan (Veracruz and Cancún), Brazil (São Paulo and Rio de Janeiro), Peru, and Cuba all come together here, sparked by influences from the West Indies and Argentina. That means the seasoning ranges from mild to very hot, and the dishes provide a lot of interesting flavors and ingredients. Ceviche in a number of intriguing variations is the house specialty. Business diners will find this restaurant a fine change of pace.

APPETIZERS, SOUPS, AND SALADS

Grouper Ceviche "Clasico" with Manzanilla Olives and Shaved Radish	ALL PHASES
Yucatan Shrimp Cocktail Ceviche with Pico de Gallo and Avocado	ALL PHASES
Golden Tomato Gazpacho with Peekytoe Crab Ceviche	ALL PHASES
Grilled Octopus Salad	ALL PHASES
Yellowfin Tuna Ceviche with Cucumber and Mango	PHASE 2

ENTRÉES

Pacific Halibut Filet with a Cilantro Crust	ALL PHASES
Bahian Style "Bouillabaisse" Mouqueca	ALL PHASES
Brazilian Braised Pork Shank "Feijoada" with Black Beans	PHASE 3

❦ The Occidental Restaurant ❧

1475 Pennsylvania Avenue, NW, Washington, DC 20004
(202) 783-1475, www.occidentaldc.com

Since 1906, The Occidental has been the favorite place for Washington's celebrities and power elite to see and be seen—it's often called "the second most famous address on Pennsylvania Avenue." The elegant dining rooms are decorated in the original style, with plenty of brass and dark wood. The cooking here is primarily traditional American, with intense, bold flavors and some interesting culinary twists; the award-winning wine list complements the menu nicely.

APPETIZERS AND SALADS

Hand-Cut Tuna Tartare	ALL PHASES
Jumbo Shrimp Cocktail with Vodka Horseradish Sauce	ALL PHASES
Maine Lobster Salad with Avocado and Passion Fruit Vinaigrette	ALL PHASES
Spring Greens Salad with Maytag Blue Cheese and Poached Pears	PHASE 2
Roasted Baby Beet and Golden Beet Salad with Goat Cheese	PHASE 3

ENTRÉES

Roasted Garlic Swordfish in a Spicy Tomato Sauce	ALL PHASES
Seared Salmon with Baby Spinach and Green Herb Sauce	ALL PHASES
Seared Maine Scallops with House-Made Kimchee	ALL PHASES
Filet Mignon in Red Wine Jus	PHASE 2
Double-Cut Pork Chop with French Green Beans and Country Mushroom Sauce	PHASE 3

SIDE DISHES

French Green Beans	ALL PHASES
Grilled Asparagus	ALL PHASES

❧ Restaurant Kolumbia ❧

1801 K Street, NW, Washington, DC 20006
(202) 331-5551, www.restaurantkolumbia.com

The stunning interior of Restaurant Kolumbia is elegant but welcoming—much like the food. The cuisine is contemporary fusion attuned to the season, and the menu changes often to best use local produce. The cooking is solidly grounded in classical French technique, but with Middle Eastern influences. In keeping with the fusion concept, dishes here often combine the ordinary with the unusual or bring together two unrelated or contrasting ingredients. The success rate is very high, making Restaurant Kolumbia a great place to dine with friends or colleagues.

APPETIZERS AND SALADS

Clam Ceviche "Casino" with Warm Sherry Vinaigrette and Parmesan Mousseline	ALL PHASES
Salad of Fava Beans, Lentils, Butter Lettuce, and Creamy Chèvre	PHASE 2

ENTRÉES

Baked Halibut with Dungeness Crab, Braised Endive, and Asparagus	ALL PHASES
Saffron-Crusted Lamb Loin over Pistou Beans with Olive Demi-Glace and Artichokes	ALL PHASES
Roasted Saddle of Rabbit with Green Olives and Rosemary Juice	PHASE 2

SIDE DISHES

Sautéed Vegetables	ALL PHASES
Broccoli Rabe	ALL PHASES
Whole Grain "Pilaf"	PHASE 2

INDEX

Underscored page references indicate boxed text.

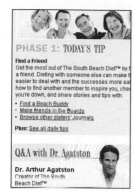

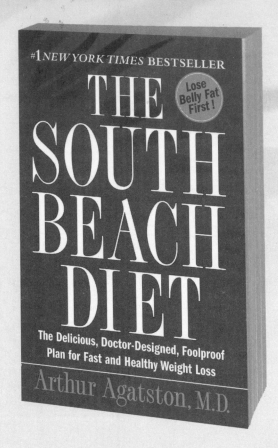